日英対訳
GMP監査チェックリスト

PIC/S GMPに基づく国内外製造所監査の勘所

著 古澤 久仁彦

じほう

本書執筆にあたって

　2016年9月に,「リスクベースによるGMP監査実施ノウハウ」をじほうから発行し,GMP監査を実施する多くの方々の参考書として活用いただいているが,これを受け「実情に合った監査員の質問集」を希望する声が寄せられるようになった。特に海外の製造所を監査するときに聞くべき項目についての困難さが,筆者の耳によく届くようになった。PIC/S GMP Guideの構成は,ICH Q7とは異なるため,「リスクベースによるGMP監査実施ノウハウ」に掲載した質問集とは別に,PIC/S GMPに基づいた対応を示す質問集が求められているのであろう。

　こうした声にお応えすべく,PIC/S GMP Guideの最新版(PE009-14)に準拠して,各章に対応する質問集を準備した。特に海外での監査にも使えるよう,質問は日本語,英語併記とした。質問内容は,できるだけ簡素な表現・言葉でまとめるように配慮した。

　今回本書では,チェックリストとして,4場面の監査を想定して,全Ⅳ章構成で質問事項をまとめた。

　　第Ⅰ章　Audit Checklist for Drug Substance（API）／原薬製造所の監査チェックリスト
　　第Ⅱ章　Audit Checklist for Finished Products／医薬品製剤製造所の監査チェックリスト
　　第Ⅲ章　Audit Checklist for Plant/Laboratory Tour／
　　　　　　プラント／ラボツアー実施のためのチェックリスト
　　第Ⅳ章　Audit Checklist on Prevention for Cross Contamination／
　　　　　　交叉汚染対策のためのチェックリスト

　第Ⅰ・Ⅱ章は,それぞれPIC/S GMP GuideのPart Ⅱ*とPart Ⅰの構成に沿った形でチェックリストをまとめ,第Ⅲ・Ⅳ章では,Annex等も含め全般的に要件を収載している。
※本書では,PIC/S GMP Guide Part Ⅱの「19. APIs FOR USE IN CLINICAL TRIALS」（治験薬）については対象としていない点に留意されたい。

　それぞれのチェックリストを自社の実情に合わせてブラッシュアップして活用し,GMP監査実施にお役立ていただきたい。

2018年8月　古澤 久仁彦

目次

本書執筆にあたって ……………………………………… i
本書の使い方 …………………………………………… vi

第Ⅰ章　Audit Checklist for Drug Substance（API）／原薬製造所の監査チェックリスト　　001

1　Introduction／導入　　002
Scope（範囲）▶002

2　Quality Management System／品質システム　　003
Principles（原則）▶003　　Quality Risk Management（品質リスクマネジメント）▶003　　Responsibilities of the Quality Unit(s)（品質部門の責務）▶004　　Responsibilities for Production Activities（生産活動の責務）▶004　　Internal audits (Self inspections)（自己点検）▶004　　Product Quality Review (PQR)（製品品質照査）▶005

3　Personnel／従業員　　006
Personnel Qualifications（従業員の適格性）▶006　　Personnel Hygiene（従業員の衛生管理）▶006　　Consultants（コンサルタント）▶007

4　Buildings and Facilities／施設・設備　　008
Design and Construction（設計・施工）▶008　　Utilities（ユーティリティ）▶009　　Containment（封じ込め）▶009　　Lighting（照明）▶010　　Sewage and Refuse（廃棄物）▶010　　Sanitation and Maintenance（清掃および保守）▶010

5　Process Equipment／工程機器　　012
Design and Construction（設計・施工）▶012　　Equipment Maintenance and Cleaning（機器の保守点検・洗浄）▶013　　Calibration（校正）▶013　　Computerized Systems（コンピュータ化システム）▶014

6　Documentation and Records／文書と記録　　016
Documentation System and Specifications（文書システムと規格）▶016　　Equipment Cleaning and Use Records（洗浄記録，使用記録）▶017　　Records of Raw Materials, Intermediates, API Labelling and Packaging Materials（出発物質，中間体，原薬，ラベル，包装材料の記録）▶017　　Master Production Instructions (Master Production and Control Records)（マスター製造指示書（製造／管理記録原本））▶018　　Batch Production Records (BPR)（バッチ製造指示書（記録書））▶019　　Laboratory Control Records（試験室管理記録）▶020　　Batch Production Record Review（バッチ製造記録の照査）▶020

7　Materials Management／原材料管理　　022
General Controls（一般管理）▶022　　Receipt and Quarantine（受領と検査）▶023　　Sampling and Testing of Incoming Production Materials（サンプリングと試験）▶025　　Storage（保管）▶025　　Re-evaluation（再評価）▶025

8　Production and In-Process Controls／製造・工程管理　　026
Production Operations（製造工程）▶026　　Time Limits（時間制限）▶027　　In-process Sampling and Controls（工程サンプリング・管理）▶027　　Blending Batches of Intermediates or APIs（中間体・原薬の異なるバッチとの混合）▶028　　Contamination Control（汚染防止）▶029

9　Packaging and Identification Labeling of APIs and Intermediates／原薬・中間体の包装，表示　　030
General（一般）▶030　　Packaging Materials（包装材料）▶030　　Label Issuance and Control（ラベルの発行と管理）▶031　　Packaging and Labelling Operations（包装・表示のオペレーション）▶031

10 Storage and Distribution／保管，輸送　　032

Warehousing Procedures（倉庫保管手順）▶032　　Distribution Procedures（輸送手順）▶032

11 Laboratory controls／試験室管理　　034

General Controls（一般管理）▶034　　Testing of Intermediates and APIs（原薬・中間体の試験）▶035　　Certificates of Analysis（分析証明書）▶035　　Stability Monitoring of APIs（原薬の安定性モニタリング）▶036　　Expiry and Retest Dating（期限切れと再テストの日付）▶036　　Reserve/Retention Samples（参考品および保管サンプル）▶036

12 Validation／バリデーション　　037

Validation Policy（バリデーション基準）▶037　　Validation Documentation（バリデーション文書）▶038　　Qualification（適格性評価）▶038　　Approach to Process Validation（プロセスバリデーションアプローチ）▶038　　Process Validation Program（プロセスバリデーションプログラム）▶038　　Periodic Review of Validated Systems（定期的照査）▶039　　Cleaning Validation（洗浄バリデーション）▶039　　Validation of Analytical Methods（分析法バリデーション）▶040

13 Change Control／変更管理　　041

Change Control（変更管理）▶041

14 Rejection and re-use of Materials／不適合品，原料の再利用　　043

Rejection（不適合）▶043　　Reworking（再加工）▶043　　Recovery of Materials and Solvents（溶媒，原料の回収）▶044　　Returns（返品）▶044

15 Complaints and Recalls／苦情・回収　　046

Complaint（苦情）▶046　　Recalls（回収）▶048

16 Contract Manufacturers (including Laboratories)／委託製造（ラボも含む）　　049

Contract manufacturers（委託製造）▶049

17 Agents, Brokers, Traders, Distributors, Re-packers and Re-labelers／代理人，ブローカー，輸入業者，流通業者，再包装・ラベル業者　　051

Applicability（適用範囲）▶051　　Traceability of Distributed APIs and Intermediates（原薬・中間体のトレーサビリティ）▶051　　Repackaging, Relabelling and Holding of APIs and Intermediates（原薬および中間体の再包装，再表示）▶051　　Stability（安定性試験）▶052　　Transfer of information（情報の移転）▶052　　Handling of Complaints and Recalls（苦情・回収の取扱い）▶052

18 Specific Guidance for APIs Manufactured by Cell Culture/Fermentation／細胞培養・発酵により製造する原薬のガイダンス　　053

Personnel（作業者）▶053　　Rooms & environment（室内および環境）▶055　　Equipment（機器）▶056　　Processes（工程）▶056　　Cell Bank Maintenance and Record Keeping（細胞バンクのメンテナンスと記録保持）▶058　　Fermentation process（発酵プロセス）▶060　　Cell Culture Process（培養工程）▶062　　Harvesting（ハーベスト）▶065　　Extraction and Isolation（抽出と分離）▶065　　Viral removal steps（ウイルス除去ステップ）▶066　　Purification（精製）▶066　　Chromatography systems（クロマトグラフィーシステム）▶067

第Ⅱ章　Audit Checklist for Finished Products／医薬品製剤製造所の監査チェックリスト　　069

1 Quality Management System／品質システム　　070

Quality Assurance（品質保証）▶070　　Product Quality Review (PQR)（製品品質照査）▶071　　Quality risk management（品質リスクマネジメント）▶071

2 Personnel／従業員　　072

General（一般）▶072　　Key Personnel（重要人員）▶072　　Training（教育訓練）▶072　　Personnel Hygiene（従業員の衛生管理）▶073

3 Premises and Equipment／施設，機器　074

Premise- general（施設 - 一般）▶074　　Premise- Production area（施設 − 製造区域）▶075　　Premise- Storage Areas（施設 − 保管区域）▶076　　Premise- Ancillary Areas（施設 − 付帯設備・施設）▶077　　Equipment（機器）▶077

4 Documentation／文書管理　080

Generation and Control of Documentation（文書の生成と制御）▶080　　Good Documentation Practices（適正文書化規範）▶080　　Retention of Documents（文書の保管）▶081　　Specifications（規格）▶081　　Manufacturing Formula and Processing Instructions - Packaging Instructions（製造指図 − 包装手順）▶082　　Manufacturing Formula and Processing Instructions - Batch Processing Record（製造指図 − バッチ記録）▶084　　Procedures and Records – Receipt（手続きと記録 − 受領）▶085　　Procedures and Records –Sampling（手続きと記録 − サンプリング）▶086　　Procedures and Records –Testing（手続きと記録 − 試験）▶086　　Procedures and Records –other（手続きと記録 − その他）▶086

5 Productions／製造　087

General（一般）▶087　　Prevention of Cross-Contamination in Production（交叉汚染防止）▶088　　Validation（バリデーション）▶088　　Starting Materials（出発物質）▶089　　Processing Operation Intermediate and Bulk products（中間体，バルク製品の製造）▶089　　Packaging Materials（包装資材）▶090　　Packaging Operation（包装工程）▶090　　Finished Products（最終製品）▶090　　Rejected, Recovered and Returned Materials（不適合，回収，返品物）▶090

6 Quality Control／品質管理　091

General（一般）▶091　　Good Quality Control Laboratory Practice（適正品質管理室規範）▶092　　Documentation（文書化）▶093　　Sampling（サンプリング）▶094　　Testing（試験）▶095　　On-going Stability Program（年次保存安定性）▶096　　Technical transfer of testing methods（試験法技術移管）▶098

7 Outsourced Activities／委託　099

General（一般）▶099　　The Contract Giver（委託者）▶099　　The Contract Acceptor（受託者）▶099　　The Contract（契約）▶100

8 Complaints and Product Recall／苦情，回収　101

Personnel and Organisation（人員と組織）▶101　　Procedures for Handling and Investigating complaints including possible quality defects（品質問題を含む苦情の取り扱いおよび調査）▶101　　Root cause analysis and Corrective and Preventive Action（原因分析と是正／予防措置）▶101　　Product Recalls and Other potential risk-reducing actions（回収とリスク低減活動）▶102

9 Self Inspection／自己点検（内部監査）　103

Principle（原則）▶103

10 Manufacture of Liquids, Creams and Ointments／液剤，クリーム，軟膏の製造　105

Premises and equipment（施設および設備）▶105　　Production（製造）▶105

11 Manufacture of Biological Medicinal Substances and Products for Human use／ヒト用生物学的医薬原薬および製剤の製造　106

Personnel（従業員）▶106　　Premises（施設）▶107　　Equipment（機器）▶108　　Starting Materials（出発物質）▶108　　Operating Principles（運用原則）▶108　　Waste Material（廃棄物の廃棄）▶108　　Biotechnological Drug product（バイオテクノロジー医薬品）▶109

第Ⅲ章　Audit Checklist for Plant/Laboratory Tour／プラント／ラボツアー実施のためのチェックリスト　111

1 Plant Tour／プラントツアー　112

APIs specific areas /activities（原薬の特定区域・活動）▶112　　Air conditional system（空調システム）▶112　　Key design parameters（設計時の要件）▶112　　Qualification of HVAC Systems（HVACシステムの適格性評価）▶113　　Qualification of HVAC Systems（HVACシステムの適格性評価）▶114　　Monitoring of HVAC Systems（HVACシステムのモニター）▶114　　Maintenance and Calibration of HVAC Systems（HVACシステムの保守点検・校正）▶114　　Documentation for HVAC Systems

（HVACシステムの文書）▶115　　Water（水）▶115　　Water quality grade（水質）▶116　　Monitoring of Warter（水のモニタリング）▶116　　Maintenance and calibration of Water Systems（水システムの保守点検と校正）▶117　　Documentation of Water Systems（水システムの文書化）▶117　　Flow of materials and personnel（動線）▶118　　Containment（封じ込め）▶118　　Design（設計）▶118　　Pharmaceutical Steam Systems, Key Design Parameters（蒸気システムの基本設計）▶118　　Pharmaceutical Gases , Key Design Criteria (compressed air)（圧縮空気ガスの設計基準）▶119　　Qualification of Utilities（ユーティリティの適格性評価）▶119　　Identify all used gases with the risk for medicinal products（使用しているガスの製品へのリスク）▶120　　Operating Systems（運転システム）▶120　　Quality Control（品質管理）▶120　　Maintenance and Calibration of the Systems（保守・校正）▶120　　Documentation of utilities（ユーティリティの文書化）▶121

2　Lab Tour in Chemical and Physical-Chemical Laboratories／化学および物理化学ラボでのラボツアー　　122

Premises（施設）▶122　　Equipment（機器）▶124　　Cleaning, Sanitation（洗浄，衛生）▶126　　Maintenance（保守管理）▶127　　Material Management（物質管理）▶128　　Water and Water Systems（水，水システム）▶130　　Sampling（サンプリング）▶130　　Handling of the samples（サンプルの取り扱い）▶132　　Personnel for Sampling（サンプリング要員）▶132　　Testing general（試験一般）▶133　　Testing of Raw Materials（原材料試験）▶133　　Testing of Intermediates（中間体の試験）▶134　　Testing of Final Products（最終製品の試験）▶134　　Stability Testing（保存安定性試験）▶135　　Validation of Test Methods（分析法バリデーション）▶136　　Handling of test results（試験結果の取り扱い）▶138　　Failures – Out of Specification (OOS) test results（規格外試験結果の取り扱い）▶138　　Failures- Retesting and Resampling（再試験・再サンプリング）▶139　　Release of test results/analytical reports/certification（出荷判定試験，分析報告書，CoA）▶139

3　Microbiological Laboratories／微生物試験室　　140

Premises（施設）▶140　　Equipment（機器）▶142　　Testing materials（試験材料）▶144　　Protective garments（更衣）▶145　　Microbiological Testing (product)（製品の微生物試験）▶146　　Microbiological testing (Environmental)（微生物試験，環境試験）▶147

第Ⅳ章　Audit Checklist on Prevention for Cross Contamination／交叉汚染対策のためのチェックリスト　　149

1　Overview on Cross Contamination／全体　　150

2　Premises, Equipment／設備・機器　　158

3　General Organisational Controls／一般組織管理　　163

4　Campaign Manufacture Organisation／キャンペーン製造　　168

5　Equipment Cleaning／機器の洗浄　　170

6　Cleaning Validation and Verification／洗浄バリデーション・ベリフィケーション　　173

7　Personnel, Training／従業員・教育訓練　　176

索引　……………………………………………………　178

本書の使い方

　本書は，GMP監査実施に際してチェックすべき項目をPIC/S GMPに基づいて紹介しています。チェックリストの見方は以下のとおりです。

❶ チェック項目	❷ チェックNO	❸ Requirement／要求事項	❹ Questions／監査時の質問例	❺ PIC/S GMP Guide Part II NO.
Scope（範囲）	I - 1	The manufacturer should designate and document the rationale for the point at which production of the API begins.	Have you designated the point at which the production of the API begins? Can a rationale be provided for this decision? Has the decision been discussed with the respective authority? Are the critical steps identified? Do you define "API Starting Materials" that is entered into the process with scientific sound?	1.2, ICH Q11
		製造者は，原薬の出発物質を特定した理論的根拠を設計・文書化せねばならない	製造所は，原薬の出発物質を特定していますか？この決定の理論的根拠を示せますか？この決定は，関係官庁と協議していますか？重要工程は特定されていますか？科学的に，プロセスにおける"原薬の出発物質"を定義していますか？	

❶監査に際してチェックする項目を記載しています。

❷本書で提示するチェックリストの通し番号です。I～IV章まで，各章ごとに番号を振ってあります。

❸PIC/S GMP Guideにおける要求事項を端的に示しています。

❹要求事項に対し，監査時に尋ねるべき質問例を記載しています。

❺関連するPIC/S GMP Guideのチャプター番号です。基本的にI章ではPart II（原薬）※，II章でPart I（製剤），III・IV章ではAnnexも含めGMP Guide全般の中で関連するチャプター番号を記載しています。

上記③～④について，英語（表内グレー部分）と日本語（表内白部分）をそれぞれ併記しております。

※ PIC/S GMP Guide Part IIの「19. APIs FOR USE IN CLINICAL TRIALS」（治験薬）については本書では取り上げておりません。

第 I 章

Audit Checklist for Drug Substance (API)／原薬製造所の監査チェックリスト

　本章で示すチェックリスト・質問例は，PIC/Sの最新GMP Guide Part II に基づいて原薬製造所を監査するためのものである。監査の範囲はGMP Guideにそろえ，1.導入，2.品質システム，3.従業員，4.施設・設備，5.工程機器，6.文書と記録，7.原材料管理，8.製造・工程管理，9.原薬・中間体の包装，表示，10.保管，輸送，11.試験室管理，12.バリデーション，13.変更管理，14.不適合品，原料の再利用，15.苦情・回収，16.委託製造（ラボも含む），17.代理人，ブローカー，輸入業者，流通業者，再包装・ラベル業者，18.細胞培養・発酵により製造する原薬のガイダンスの18項とし，治験薬については割愛している。

　本章では，監査員は原薬製造施設での品質システム，特にCAPA，リスク分析・管理に主眼を置き，また，製造所が品質の高い，安全な医薬原薬を製造することに取り組んでいるかを，実際の手順，記録を基に検証が行えるようにまとめている。チェックリストは，監査の状況に合わせ，添削を行っていただきたい。

1 Introduction／導入

まずは，GMP範囲を確認する。具体的には，出発物質の特定やその根拠，定義などを質問することが必須となる。

チェック項目	チェックNO	Requirement／要求事項	Questions／監査時の質問例	PIC/S GMP Guide Part II NO.
Scope（範囲）	I-1	The manufacturer should designate and document the rationale for the point at which production of the API begins.	Have you designated the point at which the production of the API begins? Can a rationale be provided for this decision? Has the decision been discussed with the respective authority? Are the critical steps identified? Do you define "API Starting Materials" that is entered into the process with scientific sound?	1.2, ICH Q11
		製造者は，原薬の出発物質を特定した理論的根拠を設計・文書化せねばならない	製造所は，原薬の出発物質を特定していますか？ この決定の理論的根拠を示せますか？ この決定は，関係官庁と協議していますか？ 重要工程は特定されていますか？ 科学的に，プロセスにおける"原薬の出発物質"を定義していますか？	

2 Quality Management System／品質システム

有効なシステムになっているかを確認

原薬製造における品質システムでは，リスクベースの考え方や，適切な運用体制による文書の承認・運用などがシステムとして機能しているかを確認する必要がある。
また，自己点検がしっかりと実効性をもったものになっているかも把握することが重要である。

チェック項目	チェックNO	Requirement／要求事項	Questions／監査時の質問例	PIC/S GMP Guide Part II NO.
Principles（原則）	I-2	The persons authorised to release intermediates and APIs should be specified.	The persons to release intermediates and APIs are certified and approved?	2.14
		中間体および原薬の出荷を承認する者を特定すること	中間体および原薬を出荷判定する担当者は，認定され，承認されていますか？	
	I-3	Procedures should exist for notifying responsible management in a timely manner.	Do you have Procedures for notifying responsible management in a timely manner of regulatory inspections, serious GMP deficiencies, product defects and related actions? (e.g. quality related complaints, recalls, regulatory actions, etc.).	2.18
		遅延なく，責任ある管理職に連絡する手順を持っていること	法令遵守，重大なGMPの欠陥（違反），製品の欠陥および関連する措置を適時に，責任ある管理職に連絡する手順を持っていますか？（例えば，品質関連の苦情，リコール，規制当局の措置など）	
Quality Risk Management（品質リスクマネジメント）	I-4	Quality risk management is a systematic process for the assessment, control, communication and review of risks to the quality of the active substance.	Can your Quality risk management be applied both proactively and retrospectively?	2.20
		品質リスクマネジメントは，医薬原薬の品質へのリスク評価，管理，伝達および照査のための体系的なプロセスであること	貴社の品質リスクマネジメントは積極的かつ回顧的に適用できますか？	
	I-5	To achieve the quality objective reliably there must be a comprehensively designed and correctly implemented quality system incorporating Good Manufacturing Practice, Quality Control and Quality Risk Management.	Do you including of your management establish and maintain quality systems?	2.21
		品質目標を確実に達成するためには，GMP，品質管理，品質リスク管理を組み込んだ総合的に設計され，正しく実行される品質システムを構築すること	経営層を含めて，質の高いシステムを確立し，維持していますか？	

チェック項目	チェック NO	Requirement／要求事項	Questions／監査時の質問例	PIC/S GMP Guide Part II NO.
Responsibilities of the Quality Unit(s)（品質部門の責務）	Ⅰ-6	Responsibilities of the Quality Unit(s) is to be involved in all quality-related matters.	Are your quality unit(s) involved in all quality-related matters? Do your quality unit(s) review and approve all appropriate quality-related documents?	2.30
		品質部門は，品質に関連するすべての事項に関与する責任を持つ	貴社の品質部門は，すべての品質関連事項に関与していますか？ 品質部門は，適切な品質関連文書をすべてレビューし，承認していますか？	
Responsibilities for Production Activities（生産活動の責務）	Ⅰ-7	The responsibility for production activities should be described in writing.	Do your production activities be described in writing, and involve in all quality-related matters? Do your production activities unit(s) review and approve all appropriate quality-related documents?	2.4
		生産活動の責任はすべて書面で説明されるべき	貴社の生産活動はすべて書面で説明され，また品質関連事項に関わっていますか？ 生産部門は，適切な品質関連文書をすべてレビューし，承認しますか？	
Internal audits (Self inspections)（自己点検）	Ⅰ-8	In order to verify compliance with the principles of GMP for APIs, regular internal audits should be performed in accordance with an approved schedule.	Are internal audits being performed as scheduled? Can they be substituted by third party audits? How is the frequency of internal audits a year determined? Who has responsibility?	2.50
		定期的な自己点検を，承認されたスケジュールに従って実行する必要がある	計画（スケジュール）に則して，自己点検を実施していますか？ 自己点検は，外部機関に委託できますか？ 自己点検の頻度は，年に何回ですか？ 自己点検の責任者は誰ですか？	
	Ⅰ-9	Composition of the team appropriate.	Is the composition of the audit team determined according to an SOP? Has consideration been given to: - Conflict of interest - Code of conduct - Qualifications - Independence from the area being audited Who inspects the QA function?	2.50
		自己点検の担当者は適任者を起用する	自己点検チームの構成はSOPに則して指名されますか？ 下記を考慮していますか？ ・利益相反 ・行動規範 ・適格性 ・被監査部門からの独立性 QA部門は，誰が監査しますか？	

2 Quality Management System

チェック項目	チェックNO	Requirement／要求事項	Questions／監査時の質問例	PIC/S GMP Guide Part II NO.
Internal audits (Self inspections)（自己点検）	I-10	Effectiveness of the system to plan the corrective and preventive actions, and Verification of the completion of an action.	How do you ensure that corrective actions are effective and are completed in a timely manner? How do you check the effectiveness of preventive action plan?	2.51
		是正措置および予防措置を計画するためのシステムの有効性，および措置の完了の検証	製造所は，是正措置の有効性，期間内の完了をどのように保証しますか？ 予防措置計画の有効性をどのように検証しますか？	
	I-11	The flow of information is effective.	How is the responsible management informed about the results of the audits? Do you have procedure to inform management?	2.18
		情報の伝達は効果的であること	内部監査の結果は，どのように責任ある経営層に伝達されますか？ 経営層に伝達する手順はありますか？	
Product Quality Review (PQR)（製品品質照査）	I-12	Regular quality reviews of APIs should be conducted with the objective of verifying the consistency of the process.	Are the data evaluated for the presence of trends, and are these acted upon? Are complaints, out-of-specification (OOS) and deviation investigations, reported, considered and evaluated in the PQRs? Are the PQR results used to reevaluate the expected monitoring ranges in Batch Manufacturing Records?	2.60
		定期の品質照査は，工程の頑健性・均一性に対して行われること	トレンド分析評価のデータが含まれますか？ トレンド分析は有効ですか？ 品質照査で，苦情，OOS，逸脱調査は報告がなされ，検討，評価されていますか？ 製造記録（指示）書に記載の規格値・管理値を再評価するために，年次照査結果が用いられますか？	
	I-13	Based upon the review, the validation status of a manufacturing process is evaluated and recorded.	Show me the PQR report. Do you have criteria for revalidation based on the review?	2.61
		照査に基づいて，工程のバリデーションの状況は見直され・記録されること	品質照査報告書を見せてください。 照査に基づいての再バリデーションの基準はありますか？	

3 Personnel／従業員

人員や職責等の確認

実際に生産に携わる従業員に関しては，その人員数が十分であるかといった点や，職責の規定などをまず確認する。また，従業員保護の観点から，安全性対策などについても把握する必要がある。コンサルタントについての適格性も忘れてはならない。

チェック項目	チェックNO	Requirement／要求事項	Questions／監査時の質問例	PIC/S GMP Guide Part II NO.
Personnel Qualifications（従業員の適格性）	Ⅰ-14	There should be an adequate number of personnel qualified by appropriate education, training and/or experience to perform and supervise the manufacture of intermediates and APIs.	Do you have adequate number of personnel? Do you arrange sufficiently educated, trained and certified personnel by several levels?	3.10
		製造業者は，必要な資格および実務経験を有する適切な数の人員を有すること	製造所には適切な人数の従業員が確保されていますか？ いくつかの階層別に，十分に教育訓練・認定された人員を配置していますか？	
	Ⅰ-15	To define job and prepare document of job description.	Are responsibilities of all personnel engaged in manufacture in APIs in writing available?	3.11
		業務が規定され，職務規定が文書化されていること	原薬の製造関連業務に従事する人員の職務責任は文書化されていますか？	
	Ⅰ-16	Training should be regularly conducted by qualified individuals.	Is regular training conducted? Are records of training maintained?	3.12
		教育訓練は，認定された個別の訓練者が定期的に行うこと	定例の教育訓練は行っていますか？ 教育訓練記録は保管されていますか？	
Personnel Hygiene（従業員の衛生管理）	Ⅰ-17	Personnel should practice good sanitation and health habits.	Are personnel wears clean and suitable for activity? Are there additional protective apparel where necessary?	3.21
		従業員は，衛生管理と衛生習慣を持つこと	従業員の作業着は業務に適するよう清潔に保たれていますか？ 必要であれば，追加の保護具を用いますか？	
	Ⅰ-18	To prevent cross contamination.	How is ensured that no direct contact with intermediate and APIs takes place?	3.22
		交叉汚染防止を図る	中間体・原薬に直接従業員が接触しないようになっていることをどのように担保しますか？	

3 Personnel

チェック項目	チェックNO	Requirement／要求事項	Questions／監査時の質問例	PIC/S GMP Guide Part II NO.
Personnel Hygiene（従業員の衛生管理）	I-19	Smoking, eating, drinking, chewing and the storage of food should be restricted to certain designated areas separate from the manufacturing areas.	How is ensured that no smoking, drinking, chewing and storage of food in manufacturing areas?	3.23
		喫煙，食事，飲酒，咀嚼，および食品の保管は，製造分野とは別の指定地域に限定すべき	製造域内で，喫煙，飲食，食品の保存がなされていないことをどのように担保しますか？	
	I-20	Any person shown at any time (either by medical examination or supervisory observation) to have an apparent illness or open lesions should be excluded from activities where the health condition could adversely affect the quality of the APIs until the condition is corrected.	How are personnel with infectious diseases identified? Is there a procedure in place that these persons have no product contact?	3.24
		明らかな病気や病変を有する従業員は，症状が治癒するまで原薬の品質に悪影響を及ぼす可能性のある活動から除外されるべき	どのように，従業員が罹患していないかを確認しますか？罹患者は，製品・中間体等に接触させない手順がありますか？	
Consultants（コンサルタント）	I-21	Consultants should have sufficient education, training, and experience.	Do you qualify Consultant, in advance? Are there any records of consultant: name, address, qualifications, and type of service provided by these consultants?	3.30, 3.31
		コンサルタントは，十分な経験をもち，教育訓練を受けていること	起用するコンサルタントは，前もって評価認定しますか？コンサルタントの個人情報，コンサルテーションを受ける内容は記録してありますか？	

Buildings and Facilities／施設・設備

ハードとソフト両面の確認

　汚染防止に配慮された設計になっているか，また高理活性品の専用設備化などのハード面での確認事項に加え，設備を清潔に保つための清掃スケジュールなど日常管理の面もチェックする必要がある。ここでも，GMPの基本である"文書化"がなされているかという点に着眼することが前提になる。

チェック項目	チェックNO	Requirement／要求事項	Questions／監査時の質問例	PIC/S GMP Guide Part II NO.
Design and Construction（設計・施工）	Ⅰ-22	Facilities should be designed to minimize potential contamination.	Are Buildings and facilities located, designed, and constructed to facilitate cleaning, maintenance, and operations as appropriate to the type and stage of manufacture to minimize potential contamination? Please show me the risk assessment report.	4.10
		潜在的な交叉汚染を防止できるように施設を設計すること	潜在的な汚染を最小限に抑えるために，製造のタイプと段階に応じて，適切な清掃，保守点検，および操作を容易にするために，建物や施設を配置，設計，建設していますか？ リスクアセスメントレポートを提示してください	
	Ⅰ-23	Buildings and facilities should have adequate space for the orderly placement of equipment and materials to prevent mix-ups and contamination. The flow of materials and personnel through the building or facilities should be designed to prevent mix-ups or contamination.	Have Buildings and facilities adequate space for the orderly placement of equipment and materials to prevent mix-ups and contamination? Do you design the flow of materials and personnel through the building or facilities to prevent mix-ups or contamination?	4.11, 4.13
		建物や施設には，混乱や混入を防ぐための設備や材料の整然とした配置のための十分なスペースが必要。建物や施設を通じた物質や人員の流れは，混乱や混入を防ぐように設計する必要がある	混同や交叉汚染を防ぐための設備と，材料の配置のために建物と施設に十分なスペースを設けていますか？ 混同や交叉汚染を防ぐように，建物や設備内の物／人の動線を設計していますか？	
	Ⅰ-24	Where the equipment itself provides adequate protection of the material, such equipment can be located outdoors.	Have procedures been implemented to protect the raw material, Intermediate API when exposed to each stage of the manufacturing environment (sampling, loading, unloading, etc.)?	4.12
		機器自体が適切な保護ができる場合，機器は屋外に設置することができる	原薬等が各製造段階（サンプリング，仕込み・添加，取り出しの作業）で暴露される場合は，原薬等を保護する手段が整っていますか？	

4 Buildings and Facilities

チェック項目	チェックNO	Requirement／要求事項	Questions／監査時の質問例	PIC/S GMP Guide Part II NO.
Utilities (ユーティリティ)	Ⅰ-25	Risk based qualify; DQ, PQ are required.	Are all utilities (e.g. steam, gases, compressed air, and heating, ventilation and air conditioning) qualified? Are there any procedure taken when limits are exceeded? <Challenge test were done?> Do you appropriately monitor all utility? Drawings for these utility systems approved by QA should be available?	4.2
		リスクに基づくDQ, PQが要求される	すべてのユーティリティ(蒸気, ガス, 圧縮空気, 暖房, 換気, 空調など)は検証されていますか？ 基準値を超えたときに手続きはありますか？(チャレンジテストをしましたか？) すべてのユーティリティを適切に監視していますか？ QAによって承認されたこれらのユーティリティシステムの図面は入手可能でしょうか？	
Containment (封じ込め)	Ⅰ-26	Dedicated production areas should be employed in the production of highly sensitizing materials, such as Penicillin or Cephalosporin.	Do you manufacture high sensitive products(e.g. certain steroids or cytotoxic anti-cancer agents)? Do you manufacture non pharmaceutical materials (herbicides, pesticides, etc.) in the same building/equipment as used for APIs? If there is production facilities for highly active drugs (steroids or cytotoxic anti-cancer agents) on the same premises, do you have controls been implemented to ensure to prevent cross contamination of highly toxic and validated inactivation and/or cleaning procedures, and then established and maintained?	4.40, 4.41, 4.42, 4.43
		ペニシリンやセファロスポリンなどの高感さ性物質の生産には, 専用の生産区域が必要	高理活性の医薬品（特定のステロイドや抗がん剤など）を製造していますか？ 原薬の製造に使用されているのと同じ建物／設備で非医薬品（除草剤, 農薬など）を製造していますか？ 同一敷地内で高理活性の医薬品（steroids or cytotoxic anti-cancer agents, 除草・殺虫剤）の生産設備があるならば, 封じ込める手段は整っていますか？	

チェック項目	チェックNO	Requirement／要求事項	Questions／監査時の質問例	PIC/S GMP Guide Part II NO.
Containment（封じ込め）	Ⅰ-27	Appropriate measures should be established and implemented to prevent cross-contamination from personnel, materials, etc. moving from one dedicated area to another.	Have procedures to prevent cross-contamination been established? Is the performance of these procedures being monitored? Are staffs exhibiting appropriate behavior and personal gowning procedures to prevent cross contamination?	4.42
		専用区域から別の区域に移動する人員，資材などの交叉汚染を防止するために，適切な措置を確立し，実施すること	交叉汚染防止の手順は確立していますか？ この手順の有効性はモニターされていますか？ 作業員は適切な行動をとり，交叉汚染を防止する更衣手順を行っていますか？	
	Ⅰ-28	Any production activities (including weighing, milling, or packaging) of highly toxic non-pharmaceutical materials such as herbicides and pesticides should not be conducted using the buildings and/or equipment being used for the production of APIs.	Are sensitizing, toxic and potent materials either produced in dedicated areas? Or are validated inactivation and/or cleaning procedures established and maintained?	4.43
		除草剤や農薬などの毒性の高い医薬品以外の物質の生産活動（計量，粉砕，梱包を含む）は，原薬の製造に使用されている建物や設備を使用して行わないこと	高感さ性，毒性の高い，高薬理化合物を専用設備で製造していますか？ 検証された不活性化・洗浄手順を持っていますか？	
Lighting（照明）	Ⅰ-29	Adequate lighting should be provided in all areas.	Do you monitor/evaluate the lightness at each manufacturing sites?	4.50
		すべての製造区域で，適切な照明を設置すること	各製造現場で照度を監視／評価していますか？	
Sewage and Refuse（廃棄物）	Ⅰ-30	Sewage, refuse, and other waste in and from buildings and the immediate surrounding area should be disposed of in a safe, timely, and sanitary manner. Containers and/or pipes for waste material should be clearly identified.	Is waste effectively removed from production areas (e.g. using closed systems like containers or plastic bags to prevent contamination of other areas)? Are all waste disposal systems correctly identified?	4.60
		建物やその周辺の汚水，ごみその他の廃棄物は，安全でタイムリーで衛生的な方法で処分する必要がある	廃棄物を製造区域から効果的に排除していますか（例えば汚染防止のため閉鎖系の容器・プラスチック袋を用いて）？ 廃棄システムで，廃棄物は明確に識別されていますか？	
Sanitation and Maintenance（清掃および保守）	Ⅰ-31	Buildings should be properly maintained and repaired and kept in a clean condition.	Are there documentation to define responsibility for sanitation and the cleaning schedules, methods, equipment, and materials to be used in cleaning buildings and facilities? Are these document prepared based on Risk assessment?	4.71
		建屋は適切に維持管理し，清浄に保つこと	建物や施設の清掃スケジュール，方法，設備，部材，ならびに衛生管理の責任を定めた文書はありますか？ これらの文書はリスクアセスメントに基づいて作成されていますか？	

チェック項目	チェック NO	Requirement／要求事項	Questions／監査時の質問例	PIC/S GMP Guide Part II NO.
Sanitation and Maintenance （清掃および保守）	I-32	When necessary, written procedures should also be established for the use of suitable rodenticides, insecticides, fungicides, fumigating agents, and cleaning and sanitizing agents to prevent the contamination of equipment, raw materials, packaging/labelling materials, intermediates, and APIs.	Are there any documentation for the use of suitable rodenticides, insecticides, fungicides, fumigating agents, and cleaning and sanitizing agents to prevent the contamination of equipment, raw materials, packaging/labelling materials, intermediates, and APIs? Please show me the document with QA approval	4.72
		必要に応じて，適切な殺鼠剤，殺虫剤，殺菌剤，燻蒸剤，洗浄，消毒剤を使用して機器，原材料，包装/ラベル材料，中間体，および原薬の汚染を防止するための手順書も作成する必要がある	機器，原材料，包装/表示材料，中間体，および原薬の交叉汚染を防ぐために用いられる適切な殺鼠剤，殺虫剤，殺菌剤，燻蒸剤，洗浄剤および消毒剤に関する文書はありますか？ QAが承認した文書を表示してください	

5 Process Equipment／工程機器

一定の品質をつくり出せるか

実際に原薬を製造する装置については，原材料との接触面が品質に与える影響はないか，また交叉汚染を防ぐための洗浄計画と実施状況が正しいかなどといった点が重要になる。また，常に一定の品質を生み出すことができるよう，機器の校正などが適切に行われていることも求められる。

データインテグリティも確認

装置はコンピュータ化システムが用いられることが通常になってきている。昨今話題になっているデータインテグリティ，つまりなりすましやデータ改ざんなど，データの信頼性を損なうことがないか，しっかりとセキュリティが備えられているかなども，監査において注目すべきポイントにあげられよう。

チェック項目	チェックNO	Requirement／要求事項	Questions／監査時の質問例	PIC/S GMP Guide Part II NO.
Design and Construction（設計・施工）	Ⅰ-33	Equipment should be constructed so that surfaces that contact raw materials, intermediates, or APIs do not alter the quality of the intermediates and APIs beyond the official or other established specifications.	Dose surface material to contact raw materials, intermediates, or APIs not alter the quality? Please show me the comparative report.	5.11
		原材料に接触する機器表面が，中間体または原薬の品質を変えないこと	原材料，中間体，または原薬が接触する可能性のある表面材料は，品質を変えませんか？ 適合比較レポートを示してください	
	Ⅰ-34	Major equipment and permanently installed processing lines used should be appropriately identified, Qualified.	Do you have each DQ, IQ, OQ and PQ reports, and those are approved by QA?	5.13
		主要機器および備え付けられた製造ラインは，適切に識別され，適格性を確認する	貴社は，DQ，IQ，OQ，PQの報告書を整備していますか？ それらの報告書はQAの承認がありますか？	
	Ⅰ-35	The appropriate precautions/measurements should be taken to minimize the risk of contamination.	Dose not any substances associated with the operation of equipment (e.g. lubricants, heating fluids or coolants, not contact with intermediate and/or API) contaminate?. Are food grade lubricants and oils used?	5.14, 5.15
		適切な注意・手順で，交叉汚染のリスクを最小限にすること	装置の操作に関連する物質（例えば，中間体および／または原薬と接触しない潤滑剤，熱媒体または冷却剤）は，混入しませんね？ 食品グレードの潤滑油とオイルは使用されていますか？	

5 Process Equipment

チェック項目	チェックNO	Requirement／要求事項	Questions／監査時の質問例	PIC/S GMP Guide Part II NO.
Equipment Maintenance and Cleaning（機器の保守点検・洗浄）	Ⅰ-36	Equipment maintenance schedules and procedures (including assignment of responsibility) should be established for the preventative maintenance of equipment. 機器の予防的メンテナンスのための手順を確立すべき	Are there preventive maintenance program in place? Do you follow the schedule? 予防的保守点検計画がありますか？ 計画に基づいて実施していますか？	5.20
	Ⅰ-37	Written procedures should be established for cleaning of equipment 機器の洗浄のため，文書化された手順を備えること	Are there written procedures for the cleaning of equipment in place? 洗浄・清掃手順は文書化されていますか？	5.21
	Ⅰ-38	The equipment should be cleaned at appropriate intervals 機器は適切な間隔で洗浄すること	Continuous production or dedicated production: Is there cleaned at appropriate intervals (frequency)? （連続生産もしくは専用設備の場合）適切な間隔（頻度）で清掃されていますか？	5.23
	Ⅰ-39	Non-dedicated equipment should be cleaned between production of different materials. 非専用機器では，製品切り替え時に洗浄すること	Is equipment cleaned between productions of different products? Show me acceptance criteria for residues determined 設備は，計画された異種製品製造の間で洗浄されますか？ 許容残留基準を示してください	5.24
	Ⅰ-40	Acceptance criteria for residues and the choice of cleaning procedures and cleaning agents should be defined and justified. 残留の許容基準および洗浄手順および洗浄剤の選択は，定義され，正当化すること	Do you define acceptance criteria for residues based on risk assessment from previous production? Please show the calculation procedure to define acceptance criteria for residues 前生産からの残渣の許容基準をリスクアセスメントに基づいて規定していますか？ 残渣の許容基準を定義する計算手順を示してください	5.25
	Ⅰ-41	Equipment should be identified as to its contents and its cleanliness status by appropriate means. 機器には使用目的と洗浄についての状態を表示すること	Have Equipment been identified as to its content and cleanliness status? 機器には，使用目的と洗浄（済み，前）の状態を表示していますか？	5.26
Calibration（校正）	Ⅰ-42	Critical equipments should be calibrated according to written procedures and an established schedule. 重要な機器は，決められた手順・スケジュールに準じて校正すること	Are critical equipments for intermediate and/or API qualified/ calibrated? How Do you define critical equipment? Are there written procedure in place? Is schedule of calibration followed? 中間体・原薬用の重要な機器は適正評価・校正されていますか？ どのように重要機器を選定しましたか？ その手順は整っていますか？ 校正計画を遵守していますか？	5.30

チェック項目	チェックNO	Requirement／要求事項	Questions／監査時の質問例	PIC/S GMP Guide Part II NO.
Calibration（校正）	I-43	Equipment calibrations should be performed using standards traceable to certified standards, if existing.	Does calibration done with standards that are traceable to certified standards?	5.31
		機器の校正は，場合によってトレーサブルな標準を使用して実行する必要がある	校正は，認定された基準にトレーサブルな標準で行われましたか？	
	I-44	Records of these calibrations should be maintained.	Are there records of calibration maintained?	5.32
		校正記録は，保管すること	校正記録は保管されていますか？	
	I-45	Calibration status of critical equipment should be known and verifiable.	Are calibration status of equipments easily known? How (label, electronic) to indicate of calibration status?	5.33
		重要な機器は校正の状態表示をすること	校正終了（状況）は容易に判別できますか？ どのように校正済みが表示されますか？	
	I-46	Instruments that do not meet calibration criteria should not be used.	How is ensured that instruments out of calibration are not used?	5.34
		校正基準を満たさない機器の使用禁止	校正未了の機器の使用をどのように禁止していますか？	
	I-47	Deviations on critical instruments should be investigated to determine impact.	If instruments have been shown out of calibration, are investigations performed to determine if this fact has an influence on the release of the Intermediate/API?	5.35
		重要な機器の逸脱は，及ぼす影響を調査すること	校正が不適合になった場合，校正不良が関連する中間体・原薬への影響有無を確認する調査を行っていますか？	
Computerized Systems（コンピュータ化システム）	I-48	GMP related computerized systems should be validated.	Are GMP related computer systems validated?	5.40, Annex 11-principle
		GMPに関連するコンピュータ化システムはバリデートすること	GMPに関連するコンピュータはバリデートされていますか？	
	I-49	Appropriate installation qualification and operational qualification should demonstrate.	Are IQ, OQ for Hard- and Software available?	5.40, 5.41, 5.42, Annex 11-4
		設置・可動性の確認が適正に行われていること	コンピュータの機器・ソフトの適格性は確認されましたか？	
	I-50	If an existing system was not validated at time of installation, a retrospective validation could be conducted.	Retrospective Validation for legacy systems is conducted? if not validated at time of installation,	5.41, 42
		既存のシステムは設置時に，バリデートされていない場合，回顧的に検証すること	もし，導入時にバリデーションしていないなら，既存のシステムは回顧的にバリデーションされましたか？	

5 Process Equipment

チェック項目	チェックNO	Requirement／要求事項	Questions／監査時の質問例	PIC/S GMP Guide Part II NO.
Computerized Systems（コンピュータ化システム）	I-51	Computerized systems should have sufficient controls to prevent unauthorized access or changes to data. コンピュータ化されたシステムには，不正なアクセスやデータの改ざんを防ぐための十分な管理機能を備えること	What controls are in place to prevent unauthorized access? What controls are in place to prevent changes to data? What controls are in place to prevent omissions in data? Is there a document where changes to data are recorded, who made the change, when the change was made and of the previous entry? 不正アクセスを防ぐ手段がありますか？ データ改ざん防止の手段がありますか？ データ削除防止の手段がありますか？ データの変更記録には，いつ，誰が行ったか，PCにアクセスしたかが判明する記録（文書）がありますか？	5.43, 45, Annex 11-12.1
	I-52	Written procedures should be available. 手順は文書化すること	Are there written procedures for the operation and maintenance of computerized systems available? コンピュータの運用・保守の手順が整っていますか？	5.44
	I-53	Where critical data are being entered manually, there should be an additional check on the accuracy of the entry. 重要なデータを手動で入力する場合は，正確性をさらにチェックすること	Is the entry of critical data checked by additional means (second operator or system itself)? 重要なデータは，2次照査のシステムがありますか？（第2者が行うのか，機械的か）	5.45, Annex 11-6
	I-54	Incidents related to computerized systems that could affect the quality of intermediates or APIs or the reliability of records or test results should be recorded and investigated. 中間体または原薬の品質，記録または試験結果の信頼性に影響を与える可能性のあるコンピュータ化されたシステムに関連するインシデントを記録し，調査すること	Are incidents of computerized systems recorded and investigated? コンピュータのトラブルは記録され・調査されますか？	5.46, Annex 11-13
	I-55	Changes to the computerized system should be made according to a change procedure. コンピュータ化されたシステムに変更が加えられたときは，変更管理の手順に従う	Changes to the computerized system are made according to a defined procedure? コンピュータ化システムへの変更管理は，手順に従って行われますか？	5.47, Annex 11-10
	I-56	Back-up system should be provided. バックアップを準備すること	How are data protected in cases of system breakdowns? Are there Back-up system provided? How often the company make backup? システムが停止したとき，その保護はどのようにしますか？ バックアップシステムは準備されていますか？ バックアップの頻度は？	5.48, Annex 11-7.2

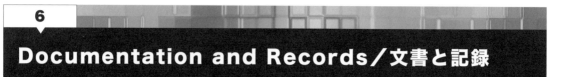

Documentation and Records／文書と記録

文書はGMP活動の根幹

他章のチェックリストでも出てきているように，文書化はGMP活動全体の根幹ともいうべきものである。そのため，製造や試験記録，洗浄など文書管理と記録保管の対象となる範囲は幅広い。すべての文書が適切に整備され，承認され，保管される手順が整っていることに始まり，"どういった状態にあるのか"を示す版管理なども要件となる。

チェック項目	チェックNO	Requirement／要求事項	Questions／監査時の質問例	PIC/S GMP Guide Part II NO.
Documentation System and Specifications（文書システムと規格）	Ⅰ-57	All documents related to the manufacture of intermediates or APIs should be prepared, reviewed, approved and distributed according to written procedures.	Written procedure in place describing preparation, review, approval and distribution of documents related to the manufacture?	6.10
		すべての原薬・中間体製造に関連する文書は，適切に照査，承認，配布されること	製造に関連する文書の準備，照査，承認，配布に関する手順が整っていますか？	
	Ⅰ-58	All documents should be controlled with maintenance of revision histories.	How do you control revision, superseding and withdrawal of documents? Is a revision history of SOP/standards/Specification maintained?	6.11
		すべての文書は，版管理を行うこと	どのように，文書の版管理，改訂を行いますか？ SOP／基準／規格の版管理の記録は保持していますか？	
	Ⅰ-59	A procedure should be established for retaining all documents.	Are procedure in place for retaining all appropriate documents? How long is Retention period specified?	6.12
		文書を保管する手順を備えること	適切な文書を保管する手順は整っていますか？ 文書の保管期間は決めてありますか？	
	Ⅰ-60	All production, control, and distribution records should be retained.	Is the retention period for APIs with expiry date: 1 year after expiry (min.)? Is the retention period for APIs with retest date: 3 years after complete distribution (min.)?	6.13
		製造，出荷，品質管理の記録は保管すること	原薬関連文書は，有効期限＋1年間は最低保管しますか？ リテストが設定されている原薬では，最後の出荷終了後，3年間は最低保管しますか？	
	Ⅰ-61	Correction should be properly done.	Are corrected entries in documents dated and signed? Are there original entries still readable?	6.14

6 Documentation and Records

チェック項目	チェックNO	Requirement／要求事項	Questions／監査時の質問例	PIC/S GMP Guide Part II NO.
Documentation System and Specifications（文書システムと規格）		訂正は適切に行うこと	文書の訂正には，適切に署名，日時が記入されていますか？ 元の記述は，確認可能になっていますか？	
	I-62	Specifications should be established and documented. 規格は制定され文書化されること	Are specifications for all raw materials, intermediates and APIs established? すべての原料，中間体，原薬の規格は確立されていますか？	6.17
	I-63	Electronic signatures should be authenticated and secure. 電子署名は，認証され，保護されること	Are electronic signatures authenticated and secure? 電子署名は，認証され，保護されていますか？	6.18
Equipment Cleaning and Use Records（洗浄記録，使用記録）	I-64	Records of cleaning and use should be properly maintained. 洗浄・使用記録は適切に維持すること	Are there records for the major equipment used, cleaning and maintenance showing the following? - date - time - product and batch number of each batch - person who performed cleaning - person who performed maintenance 重要な機器の使用，洗浄，保守記録には下記が含まれていますか？ ・日時 ・製品名，ロット番号 ・洗浄実施者 ・保守点検者	6.20
Records of Raw Materials, Intermediates, API Labelling and Packaging Materials（出発物質，中間体，原薬，ラベル，包装材料の記録）	I-65	Records should be maintained. 関連の記録を保持すること	Do you maintain records that contain next items? - name of manufacturer/supplier - identity and quantity - supplier control or identification number - number allocated on receipt - date of receipt - result of tests and conclusion derived from this - trace of use - review of labels and packaging materials showing conformity with specifications - final decision release or reject 記録には次の項目が含まれていますか？ ・製造者，販売者名 ・識別，量 ・供給者の管理もしくは識別番号 ・受領数 ・受領日 ・試験結果，その概略 ・使用履歴 ・表示，包装形態の確認 ・最終判定（適合・不適）	6.30

第Ⅰ章　Audit Checklist for Drug Substance (API)／原薬製造所の監査チェックリスト

チェック項目	チェックNO	Requirement／要求事項	Questions／監査時の質問例	PIC/S GMP Guide Part II NO.
Records of Raw Materials, Intermediates, API Labelling and Packaging Materials（出発物質，中間体，原薬，ラベル，包装材料の記録）	Ⅰ-66	Master (approved) labels should be maintained for comparison to issued labels. 発行されたラベルを検証するためマスターラベルを備えること	Are master labels maintained by Quality unit and/or responsible personnel who is independent from production? ラベルの原本管理は品質部門もしくは製造部門から独立した部門が行っていますか？	6.31
Master Production Instructions (Master Production and Control Records)（マスター製造指示書（製造／管理記録原本））	Ⅰ-67	To ensure uniformity from batch to batch, master production instructions for each intermediate and API should be prepared, dated, and signed by one person and independently checked, dated, and signed by a person in the quality unit(s). バッチ間の均一性を担保するため，中間体・原薬の製造指示書（master）を備え，品質部門が照査する	Are the manufacturing instructions (original) each of the following flow, and the quality department independently checks it? 1. Preparation 2. Description 3. Signature 4. Inspection of the QU 製造指示書（原本）はそれぞれ以下のような流れで，品質部門が独立して照査していますか？ 1.準備 2.記述 3.署名 4.品質部門の照査	6.40
	Ⅰ-68	Master production instructions should have appreciated items. マスター製造指示書には，必要な項目を含むこと	Do Master Production Instructions / record contain the following? - name of product including document reference code - complete list of raw materials - accurate statement of quantities needed or calculation of quantity - production location and major equipment to be used - detailed production instructions including sequences, ranges of parameters, sampling instructions, IPC, time limits, expected yield - instructions for storage - time limited マスター製造指示書は下記の項目が含まれていますか？ ・製品名（製品コード，認識（識別）番号） ・原材料一覧（全体） ・必要数量もしくは計算値 ・製造場所（工場名）と主要製造機器 ・シークエンス，パラメータ（許容範囲），サンプル採取指示，工程管理，時間制限，目標収量 ・保管指示 ・期限	6.41

6 Documentation and Records

チェック項目	チェック NO	Requirement／要求事項	Questions／監査時の質問例	PIC/S GMP Guide Part II NO.
Batch Production Records (BPR) (バッチ製造指示書（記録書）)	I-69	Batch production records should be prepared for each intermediate and API, and should be checked before issuance to assure that it is the correct version and a legible accurate reproduction of the appropriate master production instruction. バッチ製造記録は各中間体および原薬について準備され，発行前にチェックして，適切なマスターの正しいバージョンおよび正確な複製であることを確認する	Are batch production records checked by QU before issuance for correct version? Is it correct version and a legible accurate reproduction of the appropriate master production instruction? バッチ製造記録は，発行前に品質部門の照査がありますか？ 正しいバージョンで，適切なマスター文書の正確な複製ですか？	6.50
	I-70	Batch production records should be numbered with a unique batch or identification number. バッチ製造記録には，特異的な番号，識別できるバッチ番号を割り当てること	Dose the records have a unique batch number? 製造記録には，識別できるバッチ番号が割り当てられていますか？	6.51
	I-71	Documentation of completion of each significant step in the batch production records. バッチ製造記録は，重要工程ごとに必要項目を記載して文書を準備すること	Dose batch record contain the following? - date(s) and times (if appropriate) - identity of major equipment - identification of materials used - actual results - sampling performed - signatures of the person(s) performing the operation - IPC / laboratory test results - Actual yield(if appropriate) - Description of packaging and labels used - Deviation/investigation - Results of release testing バッチ製造記録には，次の項目が含まれていますか？ ・日付（必要に応じて時刻） ・製造機器の特定 ・使用原料の特定 ・製造実績 ・サンプリングの実施 ・作業者の署名 ・工程管理／品質管理結果 ・収率（必要に応じて） ・包装／表示 ・逸脱／調査結果 ・出荷判定試験結果	6.52

チェック項目	チェックNO	Requirement／要求事項	Questions／監査時の質問例	PIC/S GMP Guide Part II NO.
Laboratory Control Records （試験室管理記録）	Ⅰ-72	Laboratory control records should include complete data derived from all tests conducted.	Dose laboratory records contain the following? - description of sample including name, batch number or code, date when sample was taken, quantity - reference to test method - cross reference to preparation of reference standards, reagents and/or standard solutions - complete record of all raw data - record of all calculations - statement of test result if they comply with specifications - signature and date of person(s) performing the testing - signature of second person	6.60
		試験室管理記録には，行ったすべての試験に関連する記録を載せること	記録には次の項目が含まれていますか？ ・サンプルの定義，名称，バッチ番号／コード番号，サンプル採取日時，量 ・比較標準品，使用した試薬・標準液 ・生データ一式，その計算式， ・規格適合の宣言 ・試験実施者の署名 ・試験記録の確認者の署名	
	Ⅰ-73	Complete records should be maintained.	Are other records properly maintained? - modification to test method - calibration of laboratory instruments - stability testing performed - OOS investigations	6.61
		記録は保管すること	記録は適切に保管・管理されていますか？ 例えば， ・試験法の変更 ・測定機器の校正 ・実施済み／中の安定性試験結果 ・OOSの調査	
Batch Production Record Review （バッチ製造記録の照査）	Ⅰ-74	The review and approval of batch production and laboratory control records to determine compliance of the intermediate or API should be completed before a batch is released or distributed.	Is a written procedure for the handling of batch (laboratory) record review available?	6.70
		中間体または原薬のGMP遵守を照査するためのバッチ生産および品質管理記録のレビューと承認は，バッチが出荷判定または出荷する前に完了しなければならない	製造記録の照査手順は整っていますか？	

6 Documentation and Records

チェック項目	チェックNO	Requirement／要求事項	Questions／監査時の質問例	PIC/S GMP Guide Part II NO.
Batch Production Record Review（バッチ製造記録の照査）	Ⅰ-75	Batch production and laboratory control records of critical process steps should be reviewed and approved by the quality unit(s) before an API batch is released or distributed.	Are batch (laboratory) records of critical steps reviewed by the Quality Unit? Are they reviewed before the release of the API?	6.71
		製造記録・品質管理記録の重要項目は，品質部門が，出荷前に照査を終えること	製造記録・品質管理記録の重要項目は，品質部門が照査しますか？原薬出荷前に，照査は終わりますか？	
	Ⅰ-76	All deviation, investigation, and OOS reports should be reviewed as part of the batch record review.	Are all deviations, change controls, investigations and OOS reviewed as part of the batch record review?	6.72
		すべての逸脱，OOS調査は，製造記録・品質管理記録の照査の一部として行うこと	製造記録の照査には，すべての逸脱管理，変更管理，原因調査，OOS調査を含みますか？	
	Ⅰ-77	The quality unit(s) can delegate to the production unit the responsibility and authority for release of intermediates, except for those shipped outside the control of the manufacturing company.	Is the Quality Unit releasing all intermediates that are shipped outside the control of the company?	6.73
		品質部門は，製造会社の管理外に出荷されるものを除き，中間体の出荷責任と権限を，生産部門に委任することができる	製造所の管理外に出荷される中間体は，品質部門が出荷判定しますか？	

7 Materials Management／原材料管理

供給者を適切に管理

　原材料管理および供給者管理は，国内でも2013年8月の改正GMP施行通知に盛り込まれており，また今後の改正GMP省令においても要件となることが予想されている重要な要素である。製品の安定製造に向けて，原材料の入手が滞ることがないように，また品質に欠陥が起きてしまうことがないように，押さえるべき項目は複数ある。

チェック項目	チェックNO	Requirement／要求事項	Questions／監査時の質問例	PIC/S GMP Guide Part II NO.
General Controls（一般管理）	Ⅰ-78	There should be written procedures for handling of Raw materials.	Do you have procedures to contain the following? - receipt - identification - quarantine - storage - handling - sampling - testing - approval or rejection of materials.	7.10
		原材料を取り扱う手順を備えていること	次のような手順がありますか？ ・受領 ・識別 ・検査 ・保管 ・ハンドリング ・サンプリング ・受入試験 ・材料の承認または不適合判定	
	Ⅰ-79	Manufacturers of intermediates and/or APIs should have a system for evaluating the suppliers of critical materials.	Have supplier control procedures been defined and implemented? Have the following been considered in supplier control procedures? - a review of the history of supplier - completion of a questionnaire by the supplier including information about quality system, quality certifications, third party audits, site master file etc. - a supplier audit including QC labs - evaluation of samples (for new suppliers)	7.11

7 Materials Management

チェック項目	チェック NO	Requirement／要求事項	Questions／監査時の質問例	PIC/S GMP Guide Part II NO.
General Controls (一般管理)		供給者の評価，管理手順を備えていること	供給者を管理する手順が整っていますか？ 供給者を管理する手順には，次の項目が含まれていますか？ ・供給者の履歴評価 ・質問表の回答評価（品質システム，品質許可書（GMP証明書），第3者の監査結果，サイトマスターファイル） ・品質検査室を含む監査 ・サンプルの評価（新規）	
	Ⅰ-80	To sign a quality agreement.	Do you enter in the quality agreements with suppliers?	Part Ⅰ -5.28
		品質契約を結ぶこと	製造所は，（すべて）供給業者と品質契約を結んでいますか？	
	Ⅰ-81	Changes are effectively managed through the change control system.	Is the change control system used to manage changes to materials, specification and suppliers?	7.14
		（供給業者の）変更が変更管理手順で管理されていること	変更管理手順は，原料，原料規格，供給業者の変更に適用していますか？	
Receipt and Quarantine (受領と検査)	Ⅰ-82	Materials should be held under quarantine until they have been sampled, examined or tested as appropriate, and released for use.	Upon receipt and before acceptance, do you investigate each container or grouping of containers of materials; visually for correct labelling, container damage, broken seals and evidence of tampering or contamination?	7.20
		（受領した）原材料は，サンプリング・検査される，もしくは適切に試験されて使用許可が出るまで，試験中として隔離すること	受領時および受け入れ許可前に，各容器または材料の容器のグループを検査しますか？ 例えば，容器の損傷，封印の破損，改ざんまたは汚染の痕跡・証拠がないかを目視確認しますか？	

チェック項目	チェックNO	Requirement／要求事項	Questions／監査時の質問例	PIC/S GMP Guide Part II NO.
Receipt and Quarantine（受領と検査）	I -83	Validated electronic systems for material status control are acceptable. In such cases, physical segregation may not be required.	Where status control of material is required by physical location, are the locations well marked? Is access to these locations restricted to designated personnel? Where status control of material is by electronic means, is access to the electronic system restricted to designated personnel?	7.20, 10.11
		バリデートされた電子的認証・管理システムは受け入れられる。その場合，物理的な区分・隔離は特に要求されない	原料の状態・取り扱い管理が物理的に要求される場合，その場所は適切に表示されていますか？ 原料の状態・取り扱い管理が電子的である場合，電子的なアクセスは，指定された人員に限定されるシステムですか？	
	I -84	Before incoming materials are mixed with existing stocks , they should be identified as correct, tested, if appropriate, and released.	Before incoming materials (especial Bulk material) are mixed with existing stocks (e.g., material storage in silos/tank), do you investigate as correct, tested?	7.21
		既存の在庫と混合される前に，それらは正しいと判断され，適切な場合には試験され，出荷されるべき	受け入れる原材料（特にバルク品）が既存の原材料（例えば，サイロ／タンクに保管されている原材料）と混合される前に，検査していますか？	
	I -85	Receipt of Bulk material should be assurance of no cross-contamination from the tanker.	Are your assurance procedure could include one or more of the following: - certificate of cleaning - testing for trace impurities - audit of the supplier	7.22, 8.51
		受領したバルク原料は，輸送タンカーからの交叉汚染を防止する必要がある	受け入れ保証には，以下の1つ以上が含まれますか？ ・清掃証明書 ・微量不純物の試験 ・サプライヤーの監査	
	I -86	Production operations should be conducted in a manner that will prevent contamination.	If non dedicated reusable containers are used, is there evidence that they are properly cleaned? Does the cleaning procedure, and certificate of cleaning, for non-dedicated tankers cover accessory parts, including transfer hoses?	7.22, 8.51
		操作は，汚染防止を意図するように行うこと	非専用・再利用可能なコンテナを用いる際，適切に清掃されている証明がありますか？ 輸送ホース等の付属品を非専用タンクの洗浄手順・証明書に含めていますか？	

7　Materials Management

チェック項目	チェックNO	Requirement／要求事項	Questions／監査時の質問例	PIC/S GMP Guide Part II NO.
Sampling and Testing of Incoming Production Materials（サンプリングと試験）	Ⅰ-87	At least one test to verify the identity of each batch of material should be conducted.	Is each batch/container identity tested?	7.30 Annex 8-2
		材料の各バッチの同一性を検証するため，少なくとも1つのテストが実施されなければならない	各容器・バッチの確認試験を行っていますか？	
	Ⅰ-88	Sampling should be conducted at defined locations.	Do you do sampling at defined locations and with procedures to prevent contamination of the material sampled and contamination of other materials?	7.34
		サンプリングは適した環境で行うこと	各原料に適したサンプル採取環境が考慮されていますか？ サンプル採取は，サンプリングされたサンプルへの交叉汚染，他の原材料との混同を防ぐ手順で行われていますか？	
Storage（保管）	Ⅰ-89	Materials should be handled and stored in a manner to prevent degradation, contamination, and cross-contamination.	Do you have an appropriate facility for storage of material to prevent degradation, contamination, and cross-contamination? Do you identify the worst case; location in the facility? If possible, please show me your risk reduction plan.	7.40
		原材料は，分解，混入，交叉汚染を防止するように取り扱い・保管すること	分解，汚染，および交叉汚染を防ぐために，材料を保管するための適切な設備がありますか？ 施設内のワースト箇所を特定できていますか？ 可能であれば，リスク軽減計画を提示してください	
Re-evaluation（再評価）	Ⅰ-90	Materials should be re-evaluated as appropriate to determine their suitability for use.	Do you have any clear criteria to re-evaluate stored material for use of manufacturing (e.g., after prolonged storage or exposure to heat or humidity)?	7.50
		（保管されていた）原材料は，使用に適しているかを再評価する	長期間保管したり，熱や湿気にさらしたりした場合に，保存された材料を製造に使用するにあたって，再評価する明確な基準はありますか？	

8 Production and In-Process Controls／製造・工程管理

影響因子の確認

重要原料の取り扱いや，収率，重要工程の管理や担当者の認定など，実際の工程管理上影響を与える因子の確認を怠ってはならない。基本は，手順が定められ文書化されていること。また，サンプル採取する際に，そのサンプルがロットを代表していることの説明などを求めることも，場合によって必要になってくる。

チェック項目	チェックNO	Requirement／要求事項	Questions／監査時の質問例	PIC/S GMP Guide Part II NO.
Production Operations（製造工程）	I-91	Weighing and measuring devices should be of suitable accuracy for the intended use.	Are dispensing areas and equipment fit for purpose?	8.10
		計量および測定装置は，意図された用途に適した適切な精度でなければならない	調合区域と機器は目的に適合していますか？	
	I-92	The container receiving the material should be suitable and should be so identified.	Are containers suitable and appropriately labeled? Is material status controlled?	8.11
		受領した原材料の容器は適切な状態であり，それが識別できること	容器は適切なもので，ラベルが添付されていますか？ 原料の状態は，管理されていますか？	
	I-93	Critical weighing, measuring, or subdividing operations should be witnessed or subjected to an equivalent control. Prior to use, production personnel should verify that the materials are those specified in the batch record for the intended intermediate or API.	Are all critical activities witnessed or subject to equivalent controls? Do production personnel verify that materials are correct prior to use?	8.12, 8.13
		重要な計量作業は確認・検証される必要がある。また担当者は，原料に間違いがないか確認する	すべての重要な原料の計量は監視されているか，同等の管理がされていますか？ 製造の担当者は，使用に先立ち原料が間違いないかを確認していますか？	
	I-94	Actual yields should be compared with expected yields at designated steps in the production process.	Have appropriate yield ranges been set? Is the batch yield within range? For critical process steps, are deviations in yield investigated?	8.14
		期待される収率は，予想生産量と比較する	適正標準収率は定めてありますか？ バッチの収率は，規格内ですか？ 収率が逸脱した場合，調査しますか？	

8　Production and In-Process Controls

チェック項目	チェック NO	Requirement／要求事項	Questions／監査時の質問例	PIC/S GMP Guide Part II NO.
Production Operations（製造工程）	Ⅰ-95	Deviations are documented and investigated.	Are deviations documented and explained? Has an investigation been performed for critical deviations and, if necessary, corrective actions implemented?	8.15
		逸脱は文書化して報告，調査すること	逸脱は文書化され，適切に説明されていますか？ 調査は重大な逸脱に対して行われ，必要に応じCAPAを行っていますか？	
	Ⅰ-96	Process status indicated.	For each major unit of equipment is the processing status identified?	8.16
		工程の状態を表示すること	ここの重要工程機器は，適切に工程状態が表示（定義）されていますか？	
	Ⅰ-97	Reprocessing and Reworking appropriately controlled.	What systems are in place to track materials for rework, or reprocessing, and to prevent unauthorized use? Are systems prepared to prevent rework and reprocessing without permission?	8.17, 14.2, 14.3
		再加工，再処理は適切に管理すること	再加工，再処理に供される物質を追跡するにはどのようなシステムが準備されていますか？ 許可なく再加工，再処理を行わないように防止するシステムが準備されていますか？	
Time Limits（時間制限）	Ⅰ-98	Time limits for process operations, and for the storage of intermediates.	Where time limits have been set, are these being met? Are deviations documented and evaluated? How are storage conditions for intermediate held for further processing determined?	8.20, 8.21
		中間体の保管・工程管理には時間制限が求められる	時間制限が準備されている場合，その時間制限は適合していますか？ 逸脱したときは文書化し，評価していますか？ どのように，中間体の次の工程使用までの保存条件を定めていますか？	
In-process Sampling and Controls（工程サンプリング・管理）	Ⅰ-99	Written procedures available for the monitoring and control of production process.	Do written procedures exist to monitor and control the production process? Are the procedures based upon development / historical information?	8.30
		製造工程をモニター，管理するため，文書化された手順が備わっていること	製造工程をモニター，管理する手順が整っていますか？ 工程は，開発過程の情報に則していますか？	
	Ⅰ-100	Acceptance criteria appropriate to process step / stage.	Do the in-process controls and acceptance criteria become more stringent for the later processing steps?	8.31
		合格基準は，工程／ステージごとに適切であること	工程管理，合格基準は，工程が後半になるほど厳しくなっていますか？	

チェック項目	チェックNO	Requirement／要求事項	Questions／監査時の質問例	PIC/S GMP Guide Part II NO.
In-process Sampling and Controls（工程サンプリング・管理）	I-101	Critical in-process controls are documented and approved by the Quality Unit.	Has the Quality Unit given approval for critical in-process controls?	8.32
		重要工程管理は文書化され，品質部門が承認すること	品質部門は，重要工程管理を承認していますか？	
	I-102	In-process controls performed and documented by qualified staff.	Are qualified staffs performing in-process controls? Are adjustments made to processes in accordance with pre-established and validated limits? Are IPC results documented in the batch record?	8.33
		工程管理の実施と文書化は認定された人員が行うこと	認定された人員が工程管理を行っていますか？ 工程の整合・調整は，前もって確立した／検証された限度に則して行われましたか？ 工程管理の結果は，製造記録に含まれていますか？	
	I-103	Sampling Procedures documented and scientifically sound.	Are there written sampling procedures which are scientifically sound? If you assign sampling procedure; "N=$\sqrt{N}$+1", "one from one lot", please indicate scientific data that your procedure surely take representative sample of Lot.	8.34, Annex 8-4
		サンプリング手順は論理的で，文書化されていること	サンプルの採取手順は論理的で，文書化されていますか？ サンプルの採取法として$\sqrt{N}$+1，1サンプリング／ロットを採用しているならば，サンプル採取が，ロットを代表している科学的な証拠を示してください	
	I-104	In-process sampling :Prevention of contamination and assurance of the integrity of the sample.	Are sampling procedures designed to prevent contamination and ensure the integrity of the sample?	8.35, Annex 8-1
		工程サンプリングでは異物混入防止とサンプルの完全性を担保すること	工程サンプリング手順は，異物混入・汚染防止を考慮して設計され，サンプルの完全性は担保されていますか？	
Blending Batches of Intermediates or APIs（中間体・原薬の異なるバッチとの混合）	I-105	Blending of batches defined and controlled.	When you blend batches, is this process defined and controlled?	8.40
		混合するバッチを特定し，管理すること	製造所は，バッチの混合を行う際，明確に定め，管理していますか？	

8 Production and In-Process Controls

チェック項目	チェックNO	Requirement／要求事項	Questions／監査時の質問例	PIC/S GMP Guide Part II NO.
Blending Batches of Intermediates or APIs （中間体・原薬の異なるバッチとの混合）	Ⅰ-106	Only batches meeting approved specifications may be blended. 適合したバッチのみ，混合可能	Have all input batches been manufactured by the same process, been individually tested and meet specification? Is the blended batch tested for conformance with specification? すべての入力バッチを同じプロセスで製造し，個別にテストし，規格を満たしていますか？ 混合されたバッチは，規格適合試験を行っていますか？	8.41, 8.43
	Ⅰ-107	Traceability of material used in a blended batch. 混合されたバッチの履歴を残すこと	Is it possible to identify all the input batches that make up the blended batch? 混合したすべてのバッチは履歴がわかりますか？	8.44
	Ⅰ-108	Validation of the homogeneity of the blended batch. 混合後のバッチの均一性を検証すること	Is the blending operation validated to show homogeneity of the combined batch where physical attributes of APIs are critical in the dosage form? 原薬の物性（粒度，色相）が重要項目であれば，均一性を担保する混合工程のバリデーションを行っていますか？	8.45
	Ⅰ-109	Stability testing of the final blended batches should be performed. 最終混合製品の安定性に及ぼす影響を調査すること	Does the blending operation adversely affect product stability? If so, have further stability tests been performed? 混合工程は製品の安定性に影響を与えますか？ もし与えるならば，保存安定性試験を行いますか？	8.46
	Ⅰ-110	Expiry / Retest date should be based on oldest batch. 使用期限・リテスト日は，古いバッチの設定に基づく	Is the expiry/retest date of the blended batch based upon the expiry/retest date of the oldest batch in the blend? 混合品の使用期限・リテスト日は，混合する前のバッチの使用期限・リテスト日に基づいていますか？	8.47
Contamination Control （汚染防止）	Ⅰ-111	Prevention of contamination of batches by carry over from a previous batch. 前の生産バッチからの持越しによる汚染防止	Could you control the carryover of degradant and microbial contamination, that could give impact upon the established API impurity profile? (under considering the next items); - Frequency of inter batch cleaning - Environmental controls - Open processing operations 確立された不純物プロファイルに影響を与えるかもしれない分解物・微生物のキャリーオーバーを管理できますか？ 特に次の点を考慮 ・バッチ間の洗浄頻度 ・環境管理 ・開放系製造環境	8.50, 8.51, 8.52

9 Packaging and Identification Labeling of APIs and Intermediates／原薬・中間体の包装，表示

品質への影響と偽造品対策

原薬・中間体の包装においては，その資材が製品の品質へ影響を与えてはならない。適切な資材を用いたうえで，出荷ごとに表示管理し，トレーサビリティを確保するとともに，偽造品等の混入防止という観点でも注意が必要である。

チェック項目	チェックNO	Requirement／要求事項	Questions／監査時の質問例	PIC/S GMP Guide Part II NO.
General（一般）	I-112	Records should be maintained for each shipment of labels and packaging materials.	Do you maintain the record for each shipment of labels and packaging materials? Record is containing follows • receipt • examination or testing • accepted or rejected	9.12
		出荷ごとのラベル，包装資材の記録を保管すること	ラベルや梱包材の出荷ごとに記録を保持していますか？ 記録には以下が含まれていますか？ ・受領 ・検査，または試験 ・合格または不合格	
Packaging Materials（包装材料）	I-113	To grasp impact of packaging materials on product quality.	Are containers not be reactive, additive, or absorptive so as to not alter the quality of the intermediate or API beyond the specified limits?	9.21
		製品品質に及ぼす包装材料の影響を把握すること	包装資材は，不活性で，溶出・吸着がなく，原薬・中間体の品質に影響を及ぼしたり，悪化させませんか？	
	I-114	Prevention of cross contamination if containers reused.	Are there appropriate procedures to avoid mix-up and cross contamination?（under considering the next items） - cleaning - removal of labels (discard label)	9.22
		容器の再利用に伴い，汚染防止が必須である	混同，交叉汚染防止の手順が整っていますか？ 特に ・容器の洗浄 ・ラベルを取り除く（ラベルの無効化）	

9 Packaging and Identification Labeling of APIs and Intermediates

チェック項目	チェックNO	Requirement／要求事項	Questions／監査時の質問例	PIC/S GMP Guide Part II NO.
Label Issuance and Control （ラベルの発行と管理）	Ⅰ-115	The issue of labels must be controlled. 発行したラベルを管理すること	Is there an effective system for the issuing of labels? Are there logbooks for label issue? 発行したラベルの有効的な管理法は整っていますか？ ラベルの発行は記録管理していますか？	9.31
	Ⅰ-116	Security of label handling. ラベルの信頼性（偽薬対策）を確保すること	Do you control access to the label storage areas? Do you limit authorized personnel? How/who to secure label handling? Do you destroy obsolete and out-expiry date labels and record? ラベルの保管区域への立ち入りは管理していますか？ 認証した人員に限っていますか？ どのように，誰がラベルの完全性（偽造防止）を保証しますか？ 失効したラベルは記録して，廃棄しますか？	9.30, 9.33
Packaging and Labelling Operations （包装・表示のオペレーション）	Ⅰ-117	The labeling of an API must ensure traceability and provided instruction on any special transport or storage requirements. ラベルは，トレーサビリティが保証され，輸送上の特別な注意，保存条件を明示すること	If API is transferred outside the control of the manufacturer, is the name and address of the manufacturer incorporated into the label? If required, are special storage conditions incorporated into the label? 原薬が製造所の管理を外れるならば，ラベルには，製造者名・住所が記述してありますか？ 必要に応じて，ラベルに必要な特殊輸送条件が記述されますか？	9.43, 10.22
	Ⅰ-118	Effectiveness of the sealing system (counterfeit). （偽薬対策）封印は効果的であること	Has the sealing system been validated? 封印システムは検証されていますか？	9.46

10 Storage and Distribution／保管，輸送

条件・手順設定と遵守

輸送および保管においても，製品が変質することのないような適切な手順および手法が求められる。手順が文書化され，責任の所在が明確になっていることや，輸送中の品質への影響因子も含め，条件や環境について熟知している必要がある。

チェック項目	チェックNO	Requirement／要求事項	Questions／監査時の質問例	PIC/S GMP Guide Part II NO.
Warehousing Procedures（倉庫保管手順）	Ⅰ-119	Facilities should be available for the storage of all materials under appropriate conditions. 施設は，適切な環境下のすべての原材料・資材等の保管場所を備えていなければならない	Is there adequate space including specific areas for returned, rejected, quarantined materials? 返品，不適合，検査中の物資用に設けられた区域を含み，十分なスペースが準備されていますか？	4.11, 10.10
	Ⅰ-120	Appropriate storage areas. 適切な保管区域	Have the specified storage conditions been fulfilled? Show me the validation report. 定められた保管条件は，満たされていますか？ バリデーション報告書を示してください。	10.10
	Ⅰ-121	The oldest stock is used first. 古い在庫から使うこと	Are FEFO / FIFO rules met and/or effective? 先出し先入の基本を満たし，守っていますか？	7.42
Distribution Procedures（輸送手順）	Ⅰ-122	Identify personnel responsible for transport/storage. 輸送／保管の責任者を特定すること	Has the responsibility for the transport/storage been assigned? Is the assignment appropriate? 輸送と保管の責任者は決められていますか？ その指名は適切ですか？	3.11
	Ⅰ-123	APIs and intermediates should only be released for distribution to third parties after they have been released by the quality unit(s). 原薬・中間体は，品質部門の出荷判定後のみ，出荷される	Do you release APIs and intermediates for distribution to third parties only after they have been released by the quality unit(s)? あなたは品質部門の出荷承認後のみ，第三者へ出荷のために原薬および中間体を出荷しますか？	10.20
	Ⅰ-124	The transportation of the API or intermediate should follow the appropriate transport and storage conditions. 原薬・中間体の輸送は，適切な輸送・保管条件のもと行われること	How are the specified storage conditions maintained during transport? 輸送中，示された保存条件がどのように保たれていますか？	10.21

10　Storage and Distribution

チェック項目	チェックNO	Requirement／要求事項	Questions／監査時の質問例	PIC/S GMP Guide Part II NO.
Distribution Procedures （輸送手順）	Ⅰ-125	Contractor knows and follows the appropriate transport and storage conditions. 輸送業者は輸送・保管条件を熟知していること	Is the level of control over the contractor for transportation adequate? (under considering the next items) - audits for qualification - Quality agreements - questionnaire, etc. 輸送業者の管理能力は適切ですか？ ＜考慮すべき点＞ ・評価のための監査 ・品質契約 ・質問表	10.23
	Ⅰ-126	The traceability of materials and products are prepared extends to the point of first supply. 最初の中継地点以降の物・製品のトレーサビリティが準備されていること	Is there a system in place for product recall? 製品回収システムがありますか？	10.24

保管・輸送

Laboratory controls／試験室管理

OOSの頻度，保管サンプルの取り扱い

試験室の管理においては，OOSの頻度やその傾向を把握しているかといった点や，使用する標準品の適切性を確保することなどに着眼する。基本的な試験手順やサンプリング計画など，科学的根拠に基づいて行われているかどうかという点が前提となる。

チェック項目	チェックNO	Requirement／要求事項	Questions／監査時の質問例	PIC/S GMP Guide Part II NO.
General Controls（一般管理）	I -127	All specifications, sampling plans, and test procedures should be scientifically sound and appropriate to ensure that raw materials, intermediates, APIs, and labels and packaging materials conform to established standards of quality and/or purity.	Are your specifications, sampling plans, and test procedures, including changes to them prepared the draft version by the appropriate organizational unit and reviewed and approved by the quality unit(s)? All specifications, sampling plans, and test procedures for every API/Intermediate/raw material are filed? All definition of specifications, sampling plans, and test procedures have scientific sound?	11.12
		原材料，中間体，原薬，ラベルおよび包装材料が，決められた品質および／または純度規格に適合することを保証するために，すべての規格，サンプリング計画，および試験手順は科学的で適切であること	規格，サンプリング計画，テスト手順（変更を含む）は，適切な組織・部門によって草案が作成され，品質部門によって照査および承認されていますか？ すべての原薬／中間体，原材料の規格，サンプリング計画，試験手順書が準備されていますか？ 規格，サンプリング計画，およびテスト手順は，科学的根拠を持っていますか？	
	I -128	Any out-of-specification result obtained should be investigated and documented according to a procedure.	Please show the OOS report as example. How many OOS/OOT were filed in previous year? How many ration (Number of OOS/total lab test)? How to investigate cause and/or root cause?	11.15
		すべてのOOSは，手順に準拠して調査，文書化されること	OOSレポートを例として示してください。前年度，何件のOOS／OOTが提出されたのですか？ どのくらいの確率ですか（OOSの数／総試験数）？ 原因や根本原因は，どのように調査しますか？	

チェック項目	チェックNO	Requirement／要求事項	Questions／監査時の質問例	PIC/S GMP Guide Part II NO.
General Controls （一般管理）	Ⅰ-129	Each batch of secondary reference standard should be periodically requalified in accordance with a written protocol. 二次標準品は，定期的に再評価されねばならない	How many months do you requalify secondary (working) standards? Is this interval for re-qualification Scientific? 二次標準品は何カ月ごとに再認証しますか？ それは，科学的根拠に基づきますか？	11.19
Testing of Intermediates and APIs （原薬・中間体の試験）	Ⅰ-130	An impurity profile describing the identified and unidentified impurities present in a typical batch produced by a specific controlled production process should normally be established for each API. 特定の管理された製造プロセスによって製造された典型的なバッチ中に存在する，同定／未同定の不純物を含む不純物プロファイルは，通常，各原薬について規定される	Do you have procedures to review impurity profile including the identity or some qualitative analytical designation (e.g. retention time), the range of each impurity observed, and classification of each identified impurity (e.g. inorganic, organic, solvent)? Do you respect ICH guidance for reviewing impurity profile? 確認試験，定性的な指標（例えば保持時間），観察される各不純物のレンジを含んでいる不純物プロファイルの照査の手順，および同定された不純物（無機，有機，溶媒など）ごとの分類手順はありますか？ 不純物プロファイルを照査するためにICHガイダンスに準拠していますか？	11.21, 11.22
	Ⅰ-131	Appropriate microbiological tests should be conducted on each batch of intermediate and API. 中間体および原薬の各バッチに対して，適切な微生物学的試験を行うこと	When microbial quality is specified, do you conduct microbial quality test for every Batches? 微生物の規格が設定された場合，バッチごとに微生物品質検査を実施しますか？	11.23
Certificates of Analysis （分析証明書）	Ⅰ-132	Authentic Certificates of Analysis should be issued for each batch of intermediate or API on request. 分析証明書（CoA）には，必要な顧客または顧客の要件に準じて行った各テストが記載されること	Does the CoA include each test conducted according to the requirements of the necessary customers or customers? CoAには，必要な顧客または顧客の要件に従って実施された各テストが含まれていますか？	11.42
	Ⅰ-133	Where the analysis has been carried out by a re-packer or re-processor, the Certificate of Analysis should show the name, address and telephone number of the re-packer/re-processor and a reference to the name of the original manufacturer. 分析・検査が再包装業者または再処理業者によって行われた場合，CoAには，再包装業者／再処理業者の名前，住所，電話番号，および元の製造元の名前が表示されること	Do you have review CoA system issued by a re-packer or re-processor? 再包装業者・再処理業者が発行したCoAを照査するシステムを持っていますか？	11.44

チェック項目	チェックNO	Requirement／要求事項	Questions／監査時の質問例	PIC/S GMP Guide Part II NO.
Stability Monitoring of APIs（原薬の安定性モニタリング）	Ⅰ-134	A documented, on-going testing program should be designed to monitor the stability characteristics of APIs.	Do you review on-going stability test results to confirm appropriate storage conditions and retest or expiry dates? If fail of stability test, how to review storage conditions and retest or expiry dates?	11.50
		文書化されている保存安定性試験は，原薬の安定性を監視するように設計されていること	保管条件と再テストまたは有効期限を確認するために，保存安定性試験の結果を確認しますか？ 安定性試験が不適になった場合，保管条件と再テストまたは有効期限の見直し方法は？	
	Ⅰ-135	For APIs with short shelf-lives, testing should be done more frequently.	For biotechnological/biological and other APIs with shelf-lives of one year or less, do you test monthly for the first three months, and at three month intervals after then?	11.55
		保存有効期間が短い原薬に対しては，頻度高く保存安定性を評価すること	1年以下の有効期間を有するバイオテクノロジー／生物学的およびその他の原薬の場合，最初の3カ月間は毎月，その後は3カ月ごとに保存安定性の分析評価をしますか？	
Expiry and Retest Dating（期限切れと再テストの日付）	Ⅰ-136	When an intermediate is intended to be transferred outside and an expiry or retest date is assigned, supporting stability information should be available.	Do you have any expiry date for intermediates and/or conduct stability study of intermediate?	11.60
		中間体が，自社GMP管理外に輸送されるとき，有効期限・再テスト日を定めること	中間体の有効期限は設定してありますか？中間体の安定性試験を実施していますか？	
Reserve/Retention Samples（参考品および保管サンプル）	Ⅰ-137	Sufficient quantities of reserve samples should be retained.	How many samples do you stock as retention samples? If you have complaints more than two times, how to investigate Quality complaints?	11.72
		保管サンプルは，十分量保持すること	保管サンプルとしていくつのサンプルを保持していますか？ 2回以上苦情があった場合は，どのように品質苦情を調査するのですか？	

12 Validation／バリデーション

幅広い観点での確認

洗浄バリデーション，分析法バリデーション，クオリフィケーション，プロセスバリデーション等，確認すべき項目が多い部分である。それぞれに，ICHやPIC/S GMP GuideのAnnexなどで細かな要求事項が示されているため，監査においては他ガイダンスも参照しながら複合的な観点で一つひとつ確認していくことが重要となる。

特に洗浄バリデーションにおいては，原料や洗浄剤等の残渣によって品質に影響がないことを検証する必要があり，昨今では毒性学的な観点でその残留許容基準を考慮する流れにもなっているため，より広い知識が求められる。以下のチェックリストでは，基本的な確認事項を示す。

チェック項目	チェックNO	Requirement／要求事項	Questions／監査時の質問例	PIC/S GMP Guide Part II NO.
Validation Policy（バリデーション基準）	I-138	The key elements of the site qualification and validation program should be clearly defined and documented in a validation master plan (VMP).	Is the Firms validation policy documented, i.e. validation master plan?	12.10, 12.11, Annex 15-1.4
		適格性・バリデーションの重要点は，バリデーションマスタープランに明確にすること	製造所のバリデーション基準は文書化していますか？ 例えば，バリデーションマスタープラン？	
	I-139	The critical parameters/attributes should normally be identified.	Are all critical manufacturing steps defined/documented? Are all critical manufacturing steps validated?	12.11, 12.12
		重要なパラメータ／属性は，特定されること	重要製造工程はすべて明確化され，文書化されていますか？ すべての重要工程は，バリデートされていますか？	
	I-140	The validation approach adopted defined and documented.	What is the validation approach adopted? (under considering the next items): - prospective, concurrent, or retrospective - the number of process runs	12.10
		バリデーションの方法は，明確化・文書化する	バリデーションの方法は何があげられますか？ ・予測的，並行的，回顧的 ・バリデーションに使用するバッチ数	

チェック項目	チェックNO	Requirement／要求事項	Questions／監査時の質問例	PIC/S GMP Guide Part II NO.
Validation Documentation（バリデーション文書）	I-141	The results of validation must be documented.	Any identified deficiencies evaluated and documented? Are variations from the protocol documented and justified?	12.22, 12.23
		バリデーション結果は，文書化すること	バリデーションの不足分は評価され，文書化されていますか？ 計画からの差異は文書化，整合されていますか？	
Qualification（適格性評価）	I-142	Qualification (DQ, IQ, OQ, PQ) conducted for critical equipments and ancillary systems (both new and existing), for intended process, as appropriate.	Have all qualification activities been completed before process validation begins?	12.30
		重要機器と付属機器システム（新規・既存）に対して，適格に作動するかの適格性評価の実施	プロセスバリデーション開始前に，すべての適格性評価は完了していますか？	
Approach to Process Validation（プロセスバリデーションアプローチ）	I-143	All operations determined critical to the quality and purity of the API are to be validated.	What a kind of criteria are an intermediate or API to meet its predetermined specifications and quality attributes?	12.12, 12.40
		品質と純度に重要だと認定されたすべての工程は，バリデートされること	中間体／原薬が，前もって決められた規格・品質特性に適合するかは，どんな基準ですか？	
	I-144	Process validation should establish whether all quality attributes and process parameters, which are considered important for ensuring the validated state and acceptable product quality, can be consistently met by the process.	Do you identify which process parameters and quality attributes were critical or non-critical based on risk assessment? The procedure to identify is clearly documented?	Annex 15-5.7
		プロセスバリデーションにおいては，その工程により，バリデートされた状態を維持し，許容できる製品品質のために重要と考えられる品質特性と工程パラメータが，継続して適合するか否かについて確認しなければならない	工程パラメータおよび品質特性が重要であるか，重要でないかをリスク分析評価に基づいて特定していますか？ その手順は，明確に文書化していますか？	
	I-145	Results which fail to meet the pre-defined acceptance criteria should be recorded as a deviation, and be fully investigated according to local procedures.	Do you discuss/investigate any implications/deviation for the validation in the report?	Annex 15-2.8
		あらかじめ規定された許容基準に適合しなかった結果は逸脱として記録し，製造所の手順に従って完全に究明しなければならない	バリデーションに対するすべての意義・逸脱についても報告書の中で考察・調査しますか？	
Process Validation Program（プロセスバリデーションプログラム）	I-146	Process validation should confirm that the impurity profile of each API is within the limits specified.	Show me the limits specification of impurities.	12.52
		プロセスバリデーションは不純物プロファイルがそれぞれの原薬規格に適合しているかを確認すること	特定した不純物の限度規格を示してください	

チェック項目	チェック NO	Requirement／要求事項	Questions／監査時の質問例	PIC/S GMP Guide Part II NO.
Periodic Review of Validated Systems （定期的照査）	I -147	There should be a periodic review of systems and processes with respect to validation status. バリデーションの状態を尊重した定期的な照査システムと手順が整っていること	Are Product Quality Reviews used to confirm that the process under review remains validated? 製品の品質照査は，照査する工程が有効であることを確認するものですか？	12.60
Cleaning Validation （洗浄バリデーション）	I -148	Focus: multi purpose facilities and final manufacturing steps. 他品目製造設備と最終工程に注目	Are cleaning procedures validated? If not, is there any justification? Is cleaning validation directed to situations that poses the greatest risk? 洗浄工程はバリデートされていますか？もしできていないなら，対応策はありますか？ 洗浄バリデーションは一番大きなリスクを対象に向き合っていますか？	12.70
	I -149	The cleaning validation protocol should be documented. 洗浄バリデーションの計画は，文書化すること	Are documents available regarding risk assessment ? (under considering the next items): -characteristics of contaminants (e.g. toxicity, solubility, potency and stability) -equipment (product contact material and relative surface area, places difficult to clean) -process flow (purification steps, bulk size, product change over) -at the minimum, selection of product(s) which represent(s) the worst case scenario (product changeover, maximum acceptable residue limit, etc.) 次のリスクに関する文書がありますか？ ・汚染物の特性（毒性，溶解性，活性，安定性） ・機器（製品が接触する材質，比較的平面か，洗浄困難か） ・工程のフロー（精製工程，バッチの大きさ，品目切り替え） ・少なくとも，ワーストケースを代表する物質の選択（品目切り替え，最大許容残留量など）	12.71

チェック項目	チェック NO	Requirement／要求事項	Questions／監査時の質問例	PIC/S GMP Guide Part II NO.
Cleaning Validation（洗浄バリデーション）	Ⅰ-150	Cleaning procedures are to be validated.	Are the cleaning procedures routinely used in production the same as those used in the validation studies? Is cleaning routinely performed after the manufacture of the same number of batches?	12.71
		洗浄法はバリデートされねばならない	洗浄バリデーションに用いられた洗浄手順が，日常の洗浄に使用されていますか？ 洗浄の間隔（バッチ間洗浄）は同じですか？	
	Ⅰ-151	Limits for the carryover of product residues should be based on a toxicological evaluation.	Do you define limit of carryover based on risk assessment with all the supporting references? Also do you define Limits for the removal of any cleaning agents used? Do you establish acceptance criteria of carryover considering the potential cumulative effect of multiple items of equipment in the process equipment chain?	Annex 15-10.6
		製品残留によるキャリーオーバーの限度値は毒性学的評価に基づかなければならない	すべての参考文献を助けにリスクアセスメントに基づいてキャリーオーバーの限度値を設定していますか？ また，使用された洗浄剤の除去のための限度値を設定していますか？ プロセス内の複数の機器の潜在的な累積効果を考慮して，キャリーオーバーの基準を確立していますか？	
	Ⅰ-152	Analytical test methods appropriately validated.	Is the analytical test method sufficiently sensitive related to the established residue limits?	12.74
		分析法（洗浄確認）はバリデートされていること	分析法は，規定された残留基準を十分満足させる感度を持っていますか？	
Validation of Analytical Methods（分析法バリデーション）	Ⅰ-153	Analytical methods should be validated unless the method employed is included in the relevant pharmacopoeia or other recognized standard reference.	Show us documents to indicate your methods are suitable to analysis.	12.80
		分析方法は，使用された方法が関連する薬局方または他の認定された参照に含まれていない限りバリデートされること	あなたの方法が分析に適していることを示す文書を提示してください	
	Ⅰ-154	Methods should be validated to include consideration of characteristics included within the ICH guidelines on validation of analytical methods.	Do you respect ICH Q3 on method validation?	12.81
		分析方法は，ICHガイドラインに含まれる特性の検討を含んでバリデートすること	ICH Q3に準拠していますか？	

Change Control／変更管理

変更がもたらす影響

製造工程など種々の変更はよく起こり得るものであるため，適切に管理されているかどうかを確認する必要がある。手順がシステマチックに構築されており，変更の承認，実施，変更後の影響評価まで一連の流れが運用されていることを確認する。

すべての変更を一律に扱うのではなく，品質への影響度などを考慮して，重大，軽微などのように分類することで，運用にあたってのリソース配分を適切に行っているかも重要な要素となる。

チェック項目	チェックNO	Requirement／要求事項	Questions／監査時の質問例	PIC/S GMP Guide Part II NO.
Change Control（変更管理）	Ⅰ-155	A formal change control system should be established to evaluate all changes.	Do you document change control procedures? Is written procedures provided for the identification, documentation, review and approval of changes?	13.10
		すべての変更を評価するために変更管理システムを確立すること	変更管理手順は，文書化されていますか？ 文書化された手順は，変更の識別，記録，評価，承認を含んでいますか？	
	Ⅰ-156	Properly specifying the subjects for change control.	Do you manage any change on raw materials, specifications, analytical methods, facilities, support systems, equipment (including computer hardware), processing steps, labeling and packaging materials, and computer software?	13.11
		変更管理の対象を適切に指定すること	原材料，規格，分析法，施設・サポートシステム，機器（コンピュータ機器を含む），製造工程，包装表示，コンピュータのソフトウェアの変更等，すべてを対象としていますか？	
	Ⅰ-157	Changes can be classified.	Is there any classification of change proposal (i.e. Major and minor)? If to justify changes required a validated process, are there system to define the level of testing, necessary of validation, and documentation?	13.13
		変更は分類・クラス分けが必要	変更のクラス分類はありますか？（例えば重大，軽微） 変更を行うにあたりバリデーションが必要ならば，試験の程度，バリデーションの必要性，文書化を設定するシステムがありますか？	

チェック項目	チェックNO	Requirement／要求事項	Questions／監査時の質問例	PIC/S GMP Guide Part II NO.
Change Control（変更管理）	Ⅰ-158	The potential impact/risk of the proposed change on the quality of the intermediate or API should be evaluated.	Are there change control system including of validation and evaluation of equivalency?	13.13
		原薬・中間体の品質に及ぼす変更の潜在的影響／リスクは評価すること	変更管理システムには，同等性のバリデーションと評価が含まれていますか？	
	Ⅰ-159	The change proposal should be reviewed and approved by the Quality Unit.	Are all changes impacting the quality of the API/Intermediate approved by the Quality Unit?	13.12
		変更申請は，品質部門によって照査・承認されること	原薬・中間体の品質に影響がある変更は，必ず品質部門により承認されますか？	
	Ⅰ-160	When the change management ends, confirm that there is no influence (to quality) due to the change	Do you evaluate the first batches produced or tested under the change?	13.15
		変更管理が終了した際，変更による（品質への）影響がないことを確認すること	あなたは，変更後の最初のバッチ・品質試験を評価しますか？	

Rejection and re-use of Materials / 不適合品，原料の再利用

適合品と明確に識別を

不適合品となった原薬・中間体は，それとわかるように隔離することが必要になる。再加工するにおいても細かな要求事項が存在するため，それらを満たさずに再加工している場合には注意が必要である。

チェック項目	チェックNO	Requirement／要求事項	Questions／監査時の質問例	PIC/S GMP Guide Part II NO.
Rejection（不適合）	Ⅰ-161	Rejected APIs and intermediate materials shall be quarantined and recorded. The disposition of material shall be recorded.	Do procedures exist and are they adequate? How are materials identified and stored? Is a list of rejected materials maintained? Do the Certificates of Destruction for disposed materials correspond with the list of rejected materials?	14.10
		不適合になった原薬・中間体は，隔離して記録すること。これらの移動は，記録すること	（不適合品の取り扱いの）手順は整っており，適切ですか？ どのように（不適合品を）識別・保管しますか？ 不適合品のリストは整備されていますか？ 不適合品のリストと不適合品の廃棄記録は整合していますか？	
Reworking（再加工）	Ⅰ-162	OOS is defined, but Reworking is not allowed.	Is an investigation performed before a decision to rework is carried out?	14.30
		OOSが確定しただけでは，再加工は認められない	再加工実施の前に，調査は十分行いますか？	
	Ⅰ-163	The impurity profile of a reworked batch shall be comparable to routine production batches.	Are the impurity profiles of reworked batches similar to routine production batches? Are the impurity profiles of reworked batches no discrepancy after storage stability?	14.32
		再加工バッチの不純物プロファイルは，通常バッチの不純物プロファイルと同等かを確認する	再加工バッチの不純物プロファイルは通常のバッチの不純物プロファイルと近似していますか？ 再加工バッチの不純物プロファイルは，保存安定性評価後も差異はありませんね？	

チェック項目	チェック NO	Requirement／要求事項	Questions／監査時の質問例	PIC/S GMP Guide Part II NO.
Reworking（再加工）	I-164	Additional testing and test methods are required if routine test methods are found to be inadequate.	Are routine analytical methods adequate for the analysis of reworked batches? Will the methods detect additional degradant or other impurities?	14.32
		規定の試験法で不都合なことが判明すれば，追加の試験，試験法が必要	通常の分析法は，再加工バッチの分析に適していますか？ その試験法は，新たな分解物・他の不純物を検出しますか？	
Recovery of Materials and Solvents（溶媒，原料の回収）	I-165	Specifications appropriate for the intended use.	Has a rationale for solvent / material specification been documented?	14.41, 14.42
		回収品には適切な規格が必須	回収品（溶媒・原料）の規格の論理的説明は文書化されていますか？	
	I-166	To ensure that solvents meet appropriate standards before reuse or co-mingling.	If recovered solvent is to be used for multiple processes, does the specification account for the presence of contaminants introduced from other processes?	14.41
		再使用または混合の前に回収溶媒が適切な基準を満たしていることを確認する	回収溶媒が色々な工程に使用されるなら，製品間の不純物の混入の基準は算出されていますか？	
	I-167	Documents and records must be maintained.	Are relevant SOPs, batch records and CoA available? Are recovered solvents formally approved and released for use?	14.40, 14.43
		記録，文書は適切に保管すること	（回収品の）SOP，バッチ記録，CoAは整っていますか？ 回収溶媒は，使用前に正式に承認，使用許可を行いますか？	
	I-168	Identification and controls of equipment used for recovery, transportation and storage of solvents.	Is the identification of the equipment used recorded or cross referenced in the batch record? Are appropriate procedures in place to avoid mix-up and cross contamination?	14.41, 14.43, 5.21
		溶媒回収に用いる機器，輸送手段，容器は認定，管理する	バッチ記録には，使用した機器の記録，相互参照が，決められていますか？ 混同，交叉互汚染を防ぐ適切な手段が整っていますか？	
Returns（返品）	I-169	Returned intermediates or APIs should be identified as such and quarantined.	If Firm accepts returns, are the returned APIs and intermediates identified as returns and subsequently quarantined?	14.50
		返品は隔離保管すること	返品を受入れた（許諾した）場合，返品された原薬・中間体は，識別され，隔離保管しますか？	

14　Rejection and re-use of Materials

不適合品，原料の再利用

チェック項目	チェックNO	Requirement／要求事項	Questions／監査時の質問例	PIC/S GMP Guide Part II NO.
Returns（返品）	Ⅰ-170	Records of returns are maintained. If the conditions under which returned intermediates or APIs have been stored or shipped before or during their return or the condition of their containers casts doubt on their quality, the returned intermediates or APIs should be reprocessed, reworked, or destroyed, as appropriate.	Does the procedures for handling returned product require the reason for returning the product to be identified? Do Firm's records allow identification of the transportation and storage history of the product, while the product was outside Firm's control? Are the details recorded in the documentation associated with the returned product adequate and appropriate? Is returned product appropriately dispositioned (released) for reprocessing, reworking, or destruction?	14.51, 14.52
		返品は記録すること。品質に疑問がある場合，必要に応じて再処理，再加工または破棄すること	返品の取り扱いの手順では，返品と識別された製品に理由を記すことを要求していますか？ 返品対象品が貴社の管理外である間，製品の輸送および保管履歴を識別できますか？ 返品された製品に関連する文書に記録されている内容は適切ですか？ 返品は，再処理，再加工，廃棄等に適切に処理されますか？	

15 Complaints and Recalls／苦情・回収

CAPAにつなげる

苦情や回収対応の手順が定められ，迅速に対応できるよう訓練も行われていることが前提になるが，それのみならず，原因やトレンド調査に基づいて，適切な是正措置を打ち出し，改善していくことが求められる。

チェック項目	チェックNO	Requirement／要求事項	Questions／監査時の質問例	PIC/S GMP Guide Part II NO.
Complaint（苦情）	Ⅰ-171	All quality related complaints should be recorded and investigated according to a written procedure.	Is there the written procedure describing the handling of complaints?	15.10
		品質に係わるすべての苦情は手順に従って，記録・調査されること	苦情を適切に取り扱う手順が整っていますか？	
	Ⅰ-172	Complaint record and handling.	Do the complaint records include the following? - name and phone number of person submitting the complaint - complaint nature (including name and batch number of API) - date complaint is received - action taken (including person taking the action) - any follow-up, if applicable - response provided to the originator of complaint including date of response - final decision on API	15.11
		苦情の記録と取り扱い	苦情の記録には次の項目が含まれていますか？ ・苦情を申し立てた人の名前，電話番号 ・苦情の種類（製品名，ロット番号含む） ・苦情受付日 ・とるべきアクション（担当者名） ・フォローアップ（可能なら） ・苦情者への回答 ・原薬の処置法	

15　Complaints and Recalls

チェック項目	チェックNO	Requirement／要求事項	Questions／監査時の質問例	PIC/S GMP Guide Part II NO.
Complaint（苦情）	Ⅰ-173	All quality related complaints recorded and investigated according to a written procedure. 定められた手順に従って，すべての品質に関する苦情は記録・調査されること	How are complaints reported, including orally, recorded and investigated? 苦情は，口頭報告を含め，どのように調査・記録されますか？	15.10
	Ⅰ-174	Complaint records include all relevant details (date and source of the complaint, nature of the complaint, references to batch number and production date). 苦情は，日時，苦情の元，苦情の性質，関連するバッチ番号・製造日を含む関連する詳細な情報を記録する	Is the nature (fact) of the complaint correctly reported – i.e. is it possible to establish if there is a recurring problem? 苦情の性質（影響）は正確に報告されていますか？例えば再発する問題があるかを検証（確認）することができますか？	15.11
	Ⅰ-175	The complaint investigation report identifies corrective actions and follow up/preventive actions. 苦情の調査報告は，是正とその確認・予防措置を定義する	Has the impact of this complaint on other batches (other relative product) been considered? 苦情に関しては他の関連バッチ（製品）を考慮して調査しますか？	15.11
	Ⅰ-176	The final report specifies the kind of response provided to the originator of the complaint and the decision on the status of the product. （苦情）最終報告は，苦情主に提示する回答を特定，製品の処理決定を明確にする	Does the corrective action correctly address the problem, or it is focused on "customer satisfaction"? (i.e. Firm looked for the root cause of the problem, or simply "reimbursed" the originator of the complaint?) Was source of the complaint removed in an effective manner through preventive actions? 是正（案）は，正確に問題を解決するようにしていますか，それとも顧客満足度を主眼においていますか？（つまり，製造者は根本原因を調査，もしくは単純に苦情主に回答しますか？） 苦情をトリガーにして是正を通して品質向上につなげますか？	15.11
	Ⅰ-177	Complaint records and reports are evaluated in the PQRs in order to identify trends, product related frequencies, and severity. 苦情の記録・報告書は，品質照査でトレンド解析，再発率，重要度を確認するために評価されること	Are complaints correctly evaluated in PQRs? (i.e. is there any evaluation of reoccurrence and trends?) Are corrective/preventive actions managed through the change control system? 苦情は，適切に品質照査で評価されますか？（例えば，頻度，トレンドの評価） CAPAは，変更管理のシステムを通して実施管理しますか？	15.12

チェック項目	チェックNO	Requirement／要求事項	Questions／監査時の質問例	PIC/S GMP Guide Part II NO.
Recalls （回収）	Ⅰ-178	The "recalls SOP" specifies the threshold (by way of example cases, or other means) for which a recall shall be considered. The "recalls SOP" specifies who can initiate a recall, and how the recall process shall be managed. (i.e. who is to be informed, and how recalled goods are to be treated and stored)	Do you clearly define/document recall process and can you easy follow?	15.13, 15.14
		回収の手順は，回収につながる検討が必要な閾値を定めていること（回収例示など）。回収の手順には，回収の宣言責任者，回収の手順管理法が定義されること（誰が回収を通告したか，回収した製品の取り扱い・保管法）	回収の手順は，明確に文書化され，容易に行うことができますか？	
	Ⅰ-179	Recall training.	Is there training plan for recall, annually?	15.14
		回収の訓練	年次で，回収の訓練を計画しますか？	
	Ⅰ-180	The recall procedure clearly defines how to inform the regulatory authorities in the case of recall related to a serious problem.	Is there aprocedure in the procedure for requesting a request for communication and cooperation (advice / guidance) to regulatory authorities in case recovery relates to safety?	15.15
		回収の対象が，重大な事象の場合，回収の手順には明確に規制当局への連絡法を定めること	回収が安全性にかかわる場合，規制当局への連絡と協力（助言・指導）依頼の要求項が手順にありますか？	

16 Contract Manufacturers (including Laboratories)／委託製造（ラボも含む）

契約に基づいた管理

委受託関係での製造・品質確保を成功させるには，両社で契約時に取りまとめる品質取り決め事項がきちんと管理・運用されているかの確認が必要になる．とくに委託先で変更が生じた際の連絡体制，大きな変更の場合のタイムリーな情報共有と承認の流れなども監査でみるべきポイントにあげられる．

チェック項目	チェックNO	Requirement／要求事項	Questions／監査時の質問例	PIC/S GMP Guide Part II NO.
Contract manufacturers（委託製造）	I-181	To cofirm the GMP on contractors.	How is the contract manufacturer evaluated for GMP compliance? Is ensured that all contract manufacturers engaged comply with the GMP requirements of Q7?	16.10
		委託先のGMPを確認すること	委託先のGMP遵守状態を評価していますか？ すべての委託先がICH Q7を遵守しているかを保証できますか？	
	I-182	There should be a written and approved contract or formal agreement between the contract giver and the contract acceptor.	Is there a written contract (Quality agreement) with the contract manufacturer? Are the GMP responsibilities defined in detail?	16.12
		委託・受託者間で，承認された契約書が必要	委託製造先と品質契約（文書）が締結されていますか？ GMPの責任は詳細に定義されていますか？	
	I-183	To audit the contract acceptor's facilities should be permited.	Does the contract permit to audit the contract manufacturer?	16.13
		監査実施が受け入れられること	委託先が監査を受諾することを明記されていますか？	
	I-184	The contract acceptor should not pass to a third party any of the work entrusted without contract giver's permission.	Is subcontracting by the contract manufacturer excluded? If not, how is ensured that the contract giver is involved in prior evaluation of the subcontractor?	16.14
		受託側は，委託者の許可なしに委託された作業のいずれかを第三者に再委託しないこと	委託製造者による再委託は，含まれませんか？ もし否ならば，委託元はどのように，孫受けの従前評価に加わることを担保できますか？	

第Ⅰ章　Audit Checklist for Drug Substance (API)／原薬製造所の監査チェックリスト

チェック項目	チェックNO	Requirement／要求事項	Questions／監査時の質問例	PIC/S GMP Guide Part II NO.
Contract manufacturers（委託製造）	Ⅰ-185	Manufacturing and laboratory records should be kept at the site.	Are all records kept at the contract manufacturers sites? How is ensured that these are readily available?	16.15
		製造・品質管理記録は，製造場所で保管すること	すべての製造関連の記録は，委託先に保管されますか？ それらがすぐに利用可能なことをどう保証しますか？	
	Ⅰ-186	Changes in the process, equipment, test methods, specifications, or other contractual requirements should not be made unless the contract giver is informed and approves the changes.	Does the contract manufacturer have a change control system? Does the contract manufacturer have a system to inform Client of significant change? How is ensure that the contract giver is informed about all intended changes of the contract manufacturer to the process? Does the contract giver approve all changes?	16.16
		工程，製造機器，品質検査法，規格すべての委託に関する変更は，委託元に連絡され，承認が得られるまで変更されない	委託製造先は，変更管理システムを保持していますか？ 重要な情報に関して，委託元に連絡するシステムがありますか？ 工程に起こるすべての変更管理が，委託元に連絡されていることをどのように保証できますか？ 委託元は，すべての変更に承認を与えていますか？（未承認がないか）	

17 Agents, Brokers, Traders, Distributors, Re-packers and Re-labelers/代理人，ブローカー，輸入業者，流通業者，再包装・ラベル業者

トレーサビリティ

医薬品製造においては，市場環境がグローバル化する中でサプライチェーンが複雑化するケースもあろう。そうした中でも，原薬・中間体製造において関係する業者をすべて適切に評価するシステムが求められる。苦情や回収といったことも想定されるため，トレーサビリティが重要な鍵を握る。

チェック項目	チェックNO	Requirement／要求事項	Questions／監査時の質問例	PIC/S GMP Guide Part II NO.
Applicability（適用範囲）	Ⅰ-187	Relevant sections of Part II are applicable to Agents, Brokers, Traders and Distributors.	Are there qualification/approval systems for Agents, Brokers, Traders, Distributors, Re-packers and Re-labelers?	17.10, 17.11, 17.30
		GMPは代理人，ブローカー，輸入販売業者にも当てはまる	代理人，ブローカー，輸入販売業者を評価・認証するシステムがありますか？	
	Ⅰ-188	Re-packers and Re-labelers are considered as manufacturers (full compliance with Part II required).	Are there authorized Vendor list on Re-packer and Re-labeler with qualification?	17.11, 17.40
		再包装（小分け包装），再ラベル業者は，製造者として扱う	再包装（小分け包装），再ラベル業者は認定・承認された業者に含まれますか？	
Traceability of Distributed APIs and Intermediates（原薬・中間体のトレーサビリティ）	Ⅰ-189	Effectiveness of the system.	For some APIs, consider the availability and completeness of required documentation back to the original manufacturer? Are these records readily available?	17.20
		効果的なシステムが必要	原薬に関して，源製造者まで遡れるようになっていますか？そのような記録は閲覧可能ですか？	
Repackaging, Relabelling and Holding of APIs and Intermediates（原薬および中間体の再包装，再表示）	Ⅰ-190	To avoid mix-ups and loss of API or intermediate identity or purity.	Is the original expiry date, API manufacturer's name and address included on the CoA and displayed on labels?	11.4
		原薬・中間体の混同または純度の混乱および損失を回避する	元の有効期限，製造業社名，住所はCoA，ラベルに表記されていますか？	
	Ⅰ-191	Repackaging, relabelling and holding of APIs and intermediates should be performed under appropriate GMP controls.	Do procedures, records, and environmental monitoring indicate that controls are in place to avoid mix-up, contamination and cross-contamination?	17.4
		原薬および中間体の再包装，再ラベルおよび保持は適切なGMP管理下で行う	製造手順，記録，環境モニターは，混同・交叉汚染防止の管理が整っていることを示していますか？	

チェック項目	チェックNO	Requirement／要求事項	Questions／監査時の質問例	PIC/S GMP Guide Part II NO.
Stability（安定性試験）	Ⅰ-192	Stability studies to justify assigned expiration or retest dates should be conducted if the API or intermediate is repackaged in a different type of container than that used by the API or intermediate manufacturer.	Is retest or expiry date available? When an API is repacked in a different type of container, are the mandatory stability studies conducted?	17.20 17.50
		原薬または中間体が原薬または中間体製造者が使用するものとは異なるタイプの容器に再包装されている場合は，割り当てられた有効期限または再検査日を正当化するための安定性試験を実施する必要がある。	再試験日，有効期限は明らかになっていますか？ 原薬が，異なる種類の容器に再包装される際，保存安定性試験は必須ですか？	
Transfer of information（情報の移転）	Ⅰ-193	Agents, brokers, distributors, repackers, or relabellers should transfer all quality or regulatory information received from an API or intermediate manufacturer to the customer, and from the customer to the API or intermediate manufacturer.	Is the customer informed of any additional manufacturing operation carried out on behalf of Agents, Brokers, Traders, Distributors, Re-packers and Re-labelers (e.g. pulverization n, Gamma irradiation, lyophilization)? Are the original API manufacturer's name, address and the batch number(s) supplied provided to the Client? Is quality or regulatory related information exchanged between partners in a timely manner?	17.60
		すべての情報は転送される必要がある	顧客には，代理人，ブローカー，輸入販売業者に代わって外部委託業者が行う追加の製造工程が連絡されますか？（粉砕，ガンマ線殺菌，凍結乾燥など） 元の原薬に関連する情報：製造業社名，住所，バッチ番号は，契約者（顧客）に連絡されますか？ 品質・法令関連情報は，業者間で緊密に連絡されますか？	
Handling of Complaints and Recalls（苦情・回収の取扱い）	Ⅰ-194	The complaint or recall should be conducted and documented by the appropriate party.	In case of quality related problems, are Agents, Brokers, Traders, Distributors, Re-packers and Re-labelers involved? Are they informed of any investigation and actions undertaken?	17.71, 17.72
		苦情または回収は，適切な当事者によって行われ，文書化されるべき	品質上の問題が発生した場合，代理人，ブローカー，輸入販売業者，再包装（小分け包装），再ラベル業者は，当事者になりますか？ 彼らには，調査・とられたアクションが連絡されますか？	

18 Specific Guidance for APIs Manufactured by Cell culture/Fermentation／細胞培養・発酵により製造する原薬のガイダンス

Annexの内容の理解を

　PIC/S GMP Guid Part Ⅱの第18セクションでは，細胞培養・発酵により製造する原薬のガイダンスが示されている。本書ではここまで主にPIC/S GMP Guid Part Ⅱ（PE009-14）の項目とそろえる形でチェックリストを示してきたが，本セクションにおいては，より細かな要件が規定されているAnnexの内容などを広く集めることを意図して作成したため，チェック項目の文言が必ずしもGMPガイドと一致しない点に留意されたい。

　バイオ原薬関連の品質保証においては特有の要件も多いため，Annexの要求事項等をうまく拾い集め，以下に例示するチェックリストに適宜項目を添削しながら，監査する品目の特徴を考慮して進めていただきたい。

チェック項目	チェックNO	Requirement／要求事項	Questions／監査時の質問例	PIC/S GMP Guide Part Ⅱ NO.
Personnel（作業者）	Ⅰ-195	Prevention of cross contamination. 交叉汚染防止	Please show us your procedure to avoid the simultaneous handling of other living or infectious material by the same persons. Do workers pass to other areas during one working day? Show me the Log books. Do workers pass from areas with active products to inactivated products (general) areas? 同じ人が他の生体物または感染性のある物質を同時に取り扱うことを防ぐ手続きを示してください 作業者は就業日中，他の作業区域を通過することはありますか？ ログブックを見せてください 作業者は，（微生物）活性がある製品を取り扱っている区域から不活性化された製品を扱う（一般的な）区域に行くことがありますか？	Annex 2-4

チェック項目	チェックNO	Requirement／要求事項	Questions／監査時の質問例	PIC/S GMP Guide Part II NO.
Personnel（作業者）	I-196	Personnel qualifications.	Are your personnel who work in areas with active products dedicated / qualified? Do personnel have background / education appropriate to the activity? Do you have a training program (qualification/continuous)? Do they have medical checks / X-rays done regularly and relative to the risk of infection? Do you check and/or control immunological status?	Annex 2-1〜3
		人員の適格性確認	（微生物）活性がある製品を取り扱っている区域で作業する従業員は，専用人員ですか，認定されていますか？ その従業員は，活性がある製品に対する知識があり，適切に教育を受けていますか？ 教育訓練プログラム（認定／継続的教育訓練）はありますか？ 定期的に感染のリスクに関連して行われる健康診断／X線検査を従業員は受けていますか？ 免疫学的状態をチェックし，および／または管理していますか？	
	I-197	To have the concept of hygiene.	Do you have a concept of hygiene including change of clothes, masks, gloves, disinfection? Do you have emergency procedure under particular circumstances?	Annex 2-1
		衛生管理方針を有すること	衣服，マスク，手袋，消毒剤の交換など，衛生に関する基本方針はありますか？ 特定の状況下での，緊急手順を持っていますか？	

18 Specific Guidance for APIs Manufactured by Cell culture/Fermentation

チェック項目	チェックNO	Requirement／要求事項	Questions／監査時の質問例	PIC/S GMP Guide Part II NO.
Rooms & environment（室内および環境）	Ⅰ-198	To keep the facility and environmental to meet Manufacturing equipment and environmental particulate and microbial contamination should be controlled.	Do you classify the room/area to the activities, appropriately? Do you design the rooms and equipment appropriate to the activities? How do you define the pressure difference (positive, negative, sink, containment)? Do you have negative pressure areas or safety cabinets used for aseptic processing of pathogens surrounded by a positive pressure sterile zone? Do you have the rooms product dedicated? Do your HVAC systems work adequate? How to demonstrate? Do you have a separation concept of areas and rooms to avoid cross contamination for the whole company Do you have a concept of environmental monitoring? Do you monitor the pressures and/or pressure difference? Do you have Procedure to operate fumigation? Do you have any procedures and a management in case of missing of integrity and damage? Do you have a system to break dedicated area?	Annex 2-5～8
		施設・機器は製造に適した状態に維持する。特に環境機器は，交叉汚染を防止するよう管理すること	活性がある製品を取り扱っている区域/部屋を適切に分類していますか？ 活性がある製品に適するように部屋や設備を設計していますか？ 差圧（正，負，低下傾向，封じ込め）をどのように定義しますか？ 陽圧滅菌ゾーンに囲まれた病原体の無菌処理をする負圧区域または安全キャビネットはありますか？ 活性がある製品専用の部屋がありますか？ HVACシステムは適切に機能していますか？どのように証明するのですか？ 会社全体で，交叉汚染防止のための区域・部屋の分離の方針を持っていますか？ 環境モニタリングの方針はありますか？ 圧力や圧力差を監視していますか？ 燻蒸（殺菌）を行う手順がありますか？ 完全性の欠如と損害が生じた場合の手順，管理手順はありますか？ 専用エリアを開放するシステムがありますか？	

第Ⅰ章 Audit Checklist for Drug Substance（API）／原薬製造所の監査チェックリスト

チェック項目	チェック NO	Requirement／要求事項	Questions／監査時の質問例	PIC/S GMP Guide Part II NO.
Rooms & environment（室内および環境）	Ⅰ-199	Environmental control to prevent cross contamination.	Do you use animals in your facility? Do you define to permit authorized persons only to access rooms/premises to the activities strictly? How do you prevent cross contamination from air?	Annex 2-6, 7, 21, 22
		交叉汚染防止のための環境管理	施設内で動物を使用していますか？ 厳格に許可された人だけが活性のある製品を扱う部屋／区域にアクセスできることを管理していますか？ どのように吸排気からの交叉汚染を防ぐのですか？	
Equipment（機器）	Ⅰ-200	To prevent cross contamination of equipment.	Are your equipment dedicated or multi-product? Do you leave equipment in the room for cleaning? If you leave equipment in the room, do you verify the equipment would be disinfected on beforehand?	Annex 2-5〜20
		機器の交叉汚染防止	機器は専用ですか，複数製品用ですか？ 洗浄するまで機器を部屋に放置していますか？ 室内に機器が置かれているとき，使用前に機器が消毒されることを確認していますか？	
	Ⅰ-201	To prevent contamination of inactivated products by activated ones.	Do you use the same equipment used both for decontamination and sterilization? Please indicate flows of contaminated materials and equipment separated from those of sterilized ones. Do you validate effluents decontaminations inter-campaign and periodically revalidate?	18.15
		活性製品からの非活性製品への汚染防止	同じ機器を除染と滅菌の両方に使用していますか？ 滅菌済みのものから分離した，汚染された材料や装置の流れを示してください キャンペーン間の排水汚染を検証し，定期的に再検証していますか？	
Processes（工程）	Ⅰ-202	To define Batch of the active ingredient to prevent mixed-up.	Do you clearly present a batch definition to comply with the marketing authorization?	Annex 2-8
		混同防止のため，活性成分を明らかにする	承認事項に準拠するためのバッチの区別を明確に表示していますか？	
	Ⅰ-203	To have the pooling strategy.	Do you have a pooling strategy exist (intermediates and drug substance) to respect the registered details?	Annex 2-6
		貯蔵の方針があること	登録状況を尊重するための貯蔵戦略（中間体と原薬）がありますか？	

チェック項目	チェック NO	Requirement／要求事項	Questions／監査時の質問例	PIC/S GMP Guide Part II NO.
Processes (工程)	Ⅰ-204	Define and document all process parameters. すべての工程パラメータを規定し文書化すること	Do you define and document all process parameters (e.g. pH, temperature, time, flow rate)? すべてのプロセスパラメータ（例えば，pH，温度，時間，流量）を規定し，文書化していますか？	Annex 2-9
	Ⅰ-205	To maintain and monitor Environment of storage/manufacturing. 製造，保存環境を監視・監視する	Do you qualify and validate HVAC, including LAF (lamina Air Flow)? Do you qualify and validate Incubation (Temperature, RPM…)? LAF（清浄空気流）を含むHVACの適格性を検証していますか？ 培養（温度，RPMなど）の適格性を検証していますか？	Annex 2-5
	Ⅰ-206	To uniform composition of each container: aliquoting conditions. 容器，分割条件	Please indicate how to demonstrate the uniformity of pooling of cells for banking if more than one vessel used - Uniform suspension - Closure verification validation - Labelling (validated to avoid loss of information on the container) - Sampling - Reconciliation - Lot number control if pooling 2つ以上の容器が使用されている場合の細胞バンクの均一性を証明する方法を示してください ・懸濁液の均一性 ・封印の検証 ・ラベリング（容器の情報が失われないように検証） ・サンプリング ・調和性 ・プールする場合のロット番号管理	ICH Q5D-2.2.2
	Ⅰ-207	To be Freezing and storage properly. 適切に凍結保存されること	Please indicate how to demonstrate stability and/or robustness; - Time limit between aliquoting and freezing - Conditions (Temperature, time limits….) 安定性および／または堅牢性を示す方法を示してください。 ・分割と冷凍の時間制限 ・条件（温度，時間制限．）	Annex 2-29

チェック項目	チェックNO	Requirement／要求事項	Questions／監査時の質問例	PIC/S GMP Guide Part II NO.
Processes （工程）	I-208	Qualification before and after freezing (characterization, testing).	Please indicate how to qualify and test cell bank. - Identity minimum before freezing - Purity minimum before freezing - Viability minimum after freezing Do you have Dedicated freezing equipment?	Annex 2-41
		凍結保存前後での性能・性質（同等性）評価	セルバンクを検証・テストする方法を提示してください ・凍結前の分割量の最小値 ・凍結前の純度の最小値 ・凍結後の生存率 専用冷凍設備はありますか？	
Cell Bank Maintenance and Record Keeping （細胞バンクのメンテナンスと記録保持）	I-209	Access for authorized personnel.	Do you define to permit authorized persons only to access rooms/premises strictly? How do you prevent unauthorized access?	18.20, Annex 2-1
		入場制限（入室）	厳密に許可された人だけが部屋／区域にアクセスすることを許可することにしていますか？ どのようにして不正アクセスを防止しますか？	
	I-210	Maintain necessary storage and storage conditions.	Do you keep storage condition of following items to meet requirement and defined specification? - Freezer or Nitrogen tank (liquid or gas phase) - Action and alert level (corrective action procedure) and Alarm system (records, 24h link) - Contamination risk - Risk reduce plan (dedicated tanks for commercial production, map and identification of the stored containers) - Procedure on identification and indication of all containers during storage to prevent mixed-up	18.21, Annex 2-6
		求められる保管条件の維持	次の項目を，要求項と定義された規格に適合するように保管条件を維持していますか？ ・冷凍庫または窒素タンク（液体または気相） ・アクション・アラート・レベル（是正措置手順）とアラーム・システム（記録，24時間連続モニター） ・汚染リスク ・リスク低減計画（汎用品用専用タンク，貯蔵容器の位置と識別） ・混同防止のための容器の識別と表示に関する手順	

18 Specific Guidance for APIs Manufactured by Cell culture/Fermentation

チェック項目	チェックNO	Requirement／要求事項	Questions／監査時の質問例	PIC/S GMP Guide Part II NO.
Cell Bank Maintenance and Record Keeping （細胞バンクのメンテナンスと記録保持）	Ⅰ-211	Traceability.	Do you have all document/record of traceability to cell banks?	Annex 2-26
		トレーサビリティを確保すること	細胞バンクへのトレーサビリティのすべての文書/記録を持っていますか？	
	Ⅰ-212	Protection from catastrophic events.	Do you prepare the counter measurement against catastrophic events? For example; Redundancy at remote sites Back-up power Automatic liquid Nitrogen fill systems	18.21
		（重大）事故からの回復	致命的な事故に対して対応手段を準備していますか？ 例えば； ・離れた地区にある余剰物 ・バックアップ電源 ・(冷凍機へ)自動液体窒素充填システム	
	Ⅰ-213	Records of use of vials.	Do your containers no return or reused? If containers is reused, please let us have your procedure on cleaning and conform of containers for use.	18.22
		容器の使用記録を残すこと	容器は単回使用か，または再使用されますか？ 容器を再使用する場合は，容器の洗浄と確認の手順を示してください	
	Ⅰ-214	Periodical monitoring.	Do you verify containers are suitability for use, periodically?	18.15
		定期的な監視	容器が使用に適していることを定期的に確認していますか？	

チェック項目	チェックNO	Requirement／要求事項	Questions／監査時の質問例	PIC/S GMP Guide Part II NO.
Fermentation process （発酵プロセス）	Ⅰ-215	To design and maintain system to be properly.	Do you do single harvest or continuous harvest (simultaneous fermentation and harvesting)? Do you design the construction, the material and the material finish (surface, roughness, polish, weld seam processing, etc.) of the following components and fittings adequate and confirm GMP rules?: - fermenter (a open or closed contained system?) - pipe work (dead legs…) - valves, vent filters - manometers - pH - thermocouples, temperature sensors - pipes and valves for charge and discharge	18.33
		システム（設備・施設）の適切な設計と維持	単回ハーベストか連続ハーベスト（同時培養とハーベスト）か？ 次のコンポーネントおよび継手の構造, 材質および材質仕上げ（表面, 粗さ, 研磨, 溶接シーム加工など）を適切に設計し, GMP規則を確認していますか？ ・培養槽（開放系, 閉鎖系容器システム？） ・パイプ作業（デッドスペース） ・バルブ, ベントフィルター ・圧力計 ・pH ・熱電対, 温度センサー ・負荷をかける, 開放用のパイプおよびバルブ	
	Ⅰ-216	To prepare and verify Cleaning and sanitizing procedures.	Do you have a procedure to clean and sterile? Do you have the testing procedure to confirm cleanness and sterile?	18.38
		洗浄・滅菌手順の検証・準備	洗浄・滅菌する手順はありますか？ 清潔さと無菌性を確認するための試験手順はありますか？	
	Ⅰ-217	To control and specify the material and matter.	Do you have the procedure to confirm/test matters to meet requirement? Please indicate the specification and test procedures; - water - media - buffers, acids, base - cell substrates - induction agent - gases - anti foam	Annex 2-31

18 Specific Guidance for APIs Manufactured by Cell culture/Fermentation

チェック項目	チェックNO	Requirement／要求事項	Questions／監査時の質問例	PIC/S GMP Guide Part II NO.
Fermentation process（発酵プロセス）		材料と物質を管理し指定する	要求項を満たすことを確認，または／テストする手順はありますか？ 規格とテスト手順を明記してください。 - 水 - 培地 - 緩衝液，酸，アルカリ - 細胞基質 - 導入薬 - ガス - 消泡剤	
	I -218	To validate and specified all process.	Are your process campaign fermentation or continuous fermentation? Does the process follow an automated procedure? Do your system proceed to add all necessary components automatically? How do demonstrate sterility of next items?: - cell substrates - water - media - buffers - gases	18.13, 18.33
		工程の特定とバリデーション	プロセスはキャンペーン形式の発酵か連続発酵ですか？ プロセスは自動化された手順に従っていますか？ 必要な原材料は，すべて自動的に追加されますか？ どのように次の項目の無菌性を検証しますか？ ・細胞基質 ・水 ・培地，培養液 ・緩衝液 ・ガス	

チェック項目	チェックNO	Requirement／要求事項	Questions／監査時の質問例	PIC/S GMP Guide Part II NO.
Cell Culture Process （培養工程）	I -219	To prevent any contamination at Process start.	What cleaning procedure for process/equipment do you have? 1, CIP Please present us qualification and validation documentation. Do you monitor after CIP and have monitoring data, e.g. on conductivity, pH? 2 Non-CIP cleaning Please present us cleaning validation documentation How do you monitor cleanliness, and have monitoring data e.g. TOC, swabbing etc.? 3,SIP sterilizing in place Please present us qualification and validation documentation Do you monitor after SIP and have monitoring data, e.g.. on temperature logging? 4. Non-SIP Please present us Sterile validation documentation How do you monitor Sterile, and have proof of sterility, e.g. media hold test	18.53, Annex 2-8
		培養開始における交叉汚染防止	プロセス／装置のクリーニングシステムはどの種類を採用していますか？ 1. CIP（定点洗浄装置） 洗浄バリデーション文書を提示してください あなたはCIP後にプロセス装置の洗浄度を検証していますか？ 監視データを持っていますか？（伝導率，pHなど） 2. 非CIP洗浄 洗浄バリデーション文書を提示してください あなたは洗浄後にプロセス装置の清浄度を検証していますか？ 監視データを持っていますか？（TOC，スワブなど） 3. SIP滅菌 滅菌バリデーション文書を提示してください あなたはSIP後に殺菌効率を監視し，例えば温度記録などの監視データを持っていますか？ 4. 非SIP 無菌バリデーション文書を提示してください あなたはどのように無菌状態を監視し，無菌性の証拠を持っていますか？（微生物増殖試験など）	18.42

18 Specific Guidance for APIs Manufactured by Cell culture/Fermentation

チェック項目	チェックNO	Requirement／要求事項	Questions／監査時の質問例	PIC/S GMP Guide Part II NO.
Cell Culture Process（培養工程）	Ⅰ-220	To ensure inoculation without cross contamination.	Do you have information on seed culture/cell bank management? Who produce the cell substrate? Please indicate Vendor. Do you have procedure of expansion of culture; e.g. in pre culture /intermediate fermenter or main fermenter? Does Vendor have an inoculation procedure in place? Does Vendor do risk assessment of contamination during inoculation? Does Vendor test bioburden of seed material? Does Vendor test endotoxins of seed material? Does Vendor control the virus content of seed material?	Annex 2-26
		交叉汚染を防止しての接種	種培養／細胞バンク管理に関する情報はありますか？ 誰が細胞基質を供給するのですか？ 供給者を示してください あなたは拡大培養；例えば 前培養／中間発酵槽または主発酵槽での手順を持っていますか？ 供給者は，施設内に接種手順を備えていますか？ 供給者は接種中に汚染のリスク評価をしていますか？ 供給者はシードのバイオバーデンを試験していますか？ 供給者はシードのエンドトキシンを試験していますか？ 供給者はシード材料のウイルス含有量を制御していますか？	

チェック項目	チェックNO	Requirement／要求事項	Questions／監査時の質問例	PIC/S GMP Guide Part II NO.
Cell Culture Process（培養工程）	I -221	To prepare and ensure Media, properly.	Do you do a growth promotion test from batch to batch? Do you have any protocols that all components are provided in the correct quantity and quality (components of animal origin: assessed for their TSE risk)? Do you produce media directly in the fermenter or produced in a media formulation tank? Do you fill media from an external source, e.g. media bag, supplier container? Do you have data that the media transfer does not affect media sterility? Do you have procedure to sterile media? Do you have data the sterility of the medium?	Annex 2-30
		培養（培地）液の適切な調整	バッチ間の成長促進テストを行っていますか？ すべての成分が正しい量と品質で提供されるというプロトコールを持っていますか？（動物起源の成分：TSEリスクについて評価されていますか） 発酵槽内で培養液を直接調整しますか？ 培養液調整タンクで調整しますか？ 外部容器から培養液を添加しますか？ 例えば，メディアバッグ，サプライヤーコンテナ？ 培地移送が，培養液の無菌性に影響しないというデータがありますか？ 培養液を滅菌する手順はありますか？ 培養液の無菌性データがありますか？	

18 Specific Guidance for APIs Manufactured by Cell culture/Fermentation

チェック項目	チェックNO	Requirement／要求事項	Questions／監査時の質問例	PIC/S GMP Guide Part II NO.
Harvesting（ハーベスト）	Ⅰ-222	Harvesting steps, either to remove cells or cellular components or to collect cellular components after disruption, should be performed in equipment and areas designed to minimize the risk of contamination.ting, Isolation and Purification.	Do you have any data that harvesting does not have a risk of contamination? Do you monitor all critical operation parameters during process as: - process time - temperature - pH - pO_2 - pCO_2 - pressure - agitation rates - addition of gases - addition of buffers, acids, lye's (alkali) - bioburden - viral content - endotoxins - viscosity	18.33
		汚染の危険性を最小限に抑えるように設計された装置および区域で，細胞または細胞成分を除去するか，または細胞崩壊後に細胞成分を収集するための収穫工程を実施すべき	ハーベストに汚染の危険性がないというデータがありますか？ プロセス中のすべての重要な作業パラメータを次のように監視していますか？ ・プロセス時間 ・温度 ・pH ・pO_2 ・pCO_2 ・圧力 ・撹拌速度 ・ガスの添加 ・バッファー，酸，アルカリの添加 ・バイオバーデン ・ウイルスの量 ・エンドトキシン ・粘度	
Extraction and Isolation（抽出と分離）	Ⅰ-223	Equipment ; Centrifugation, Filtration, Precipitation.	In the case of Aerosol formation, What is the filter life time and how is it assessed of life span?	Annex 2-16
		機器;遠心分離，フィルターろ過，沈殿	エアゾル形成の場合，フィルターの寿命はどのくらいで，寿命の評価方法は？	

チェック項目	チェックNO	Requirement／要求事項	Questions／監査時の質問例	PIC/S GMP Guide Part II NO.
Extraction and isolation（抽出と分離）	Ⅰ-224	To ensure facility and equipment to be clean, sterile to prevent contamination.	How is the equipment cleaned and how do you validate? Do you specify analytical method for product by product? Do you validate analytical method? Do you define holding times of dirty and clean equipment, and the times are covered by cleaning validation studies?	18.34
		交叉汚染防止のため，装置機器は洗浄殺菌されること	どのように装置を洗浄し，どのように洗浄の妥当性を確認しますか？製品ごとに分析方法を採用していますか？分析方法を検証していますか？機器のダーティー／クリーン保持時間を決めていますか？	
Viral removal steps（ウイルス除去ステップ）	Ⅰ-225	Process and environment; Process parameters should be specified and verified.	Do you operate critical process steps within their validated parameters?	18.33
		工程環境管理：工程パラメーターは特定され，検証される	検証されたパラメータの範囲内で重要なプロセスステップを操作していますか？	
	Ⅰ-226	To define precautions to prevent viral contamination.	Do you perform pre and post viral removal steps in separated areas with separate air handling units? Do you adapt the dedicated equipment to pre and post virus removal steps? Do workers pass from pre viral to post viral areas?	Annex 2-41
		ウイルスの交叉汚染対策	別々の加圧装置を備え，隔離された領域でウイルス除去の前後の操作を行いますか？専用の装置をウイルス除去の前後に使用しますか？従業員はウイルス除去前の作業区域からウイルス除去後の作業区域を通過しますか？	
Purification（精製）	Ⅰ-227	To specify incoming acceptance criteria of Column resins.	Do you test resins regarding: -Chemical/biological aspects -Physical aspects -Functional aspects	18.44
		クロマト樹脂の受け入れ検査	樹脂に関する以下のテストを行っていますか？ - 化学/生物学的 - 物理的 - 機能的	

18 Specific Guidance for APIs Manufactured by Cell culture/Fermentation

チェック項目	チェックNO	Requirement／要求事項	Questions／監査時の質問例	PIC/S GMP Guide Part II NO.
Purification（精製）	Ⅰ-228	To specify Performance of Column resins.	How do you define life time of resins/maximum number of runs? And What do you refer to? Do you perform HETP and asymmetric measurements? Do you test leachable teste? Do you confirm consistency of purification profiles as performance criteria? Or Do you adapt resins is dedicated to one manufacturing step of one product?	18.44
		クロマト樹脂の性能確認	どのように樹脂の寿命／最大使用回数を決めますか？ 何を参照していますか？ HETPと非対称測定を行いますか？ 漏出テストしますか？ 精製プロファイルの一貫性を性能基準として確認していますか？ または 樹脂は，1つの製品の1つの製造工程専用にさせていますか？	
Chromatography systems（クロマトグラフィーシステム）	Ⅰ-229	Column packing.	How do you calculate the size of the column resin volume? Do you define and/or study the flow and pressure during packing?	5.10
		カラム充填	どのようにしてカラム樹脂の体積を計算しますか？ 充填中の流れと圧力を設定，または調査していますか？	
	Ⅰ-230	Regular maintenance.	Do you inspect and replace of parts as preventive maintenance? How do you inspect resin/column; e.g. visual inspection of resin or other check of the column pressure?	5.20
		定期的保守を行うこと	予防メンテナンスとして部品の検査と交換を行いますか？ あなたはどのようにしてカラム／樹脂を検査しますか？ 例えば 樹脂の目視検査またはカラム圧力のチェック？	
	Ⅰ-231	Cleaning and storage.	Do you document cleaning procedure and used cleaning agents? What are the storage conditions of column/resin? Please let us conditions; e.g. temperature, time, storage solutions	5.21, 5.2
		洗浄と保管を適切に行うこと	洗浄手順を文書化していますか，洗浄剤を使用しましたか？ カラム／樹脂の保管条件は何ですか？ 条件を教えてください。例えば温度，時間，保管充填液？	

チェック項目	チェックNO	Requirement／要求事項	Questions／監査時の質問例	PIC/S GMP Guide Part II NO.
Chromatography systems （クロマトグラフィーシステム）	Ⅰ-232	Operation instruction.	Do you document the procedures; e.g. preparation, use and dismantling of the column system? Do you define specifications for critical parameters e.g. linear liquid flow, column bed height, gradient slope, temperature)?	6.10
		作業指示	手順を文書化していますか？ 例えば カラムシステムの準備，使用，および分解に関して重要なパラメータの規格を定義していますか？（直線流，カラムベッド高，勾配，温度）	

第 II 章

Audit Checklist for Finished Products／医薬品製剤製造所の監査チェックリスト

　本章で示すチェックリスト・質問例は，PIC/Sの最新版のGMP Guide Part Iに基づいて医薬品製剤製造所を監査するためのものである。監査の範囲はGMP Guideにそろえ，1.品質システム，2.従業員，3.施設，機器，4.文書管理，5.製造，6.品質管理，7.委託，8.苦情，回収，9.自己点検（内部監査）とし，さらにAnnexの内容に基づいて10.液剤，クリーム，軟膏の製造，11.ヒト用生物学的医薬原薬および製剤の製造を加えて11項のチェックリストとした。例が少ない「液剤，クリーム，軟膏」ならびに「生物由来製品・無菌製剤」に関しては，独立した項を設けて監査員の役に立つようにしているため，PIC/S GMP Guide Part Iに対応した内容になっているが，チャプター番号が必ずしも同一になっていない点はご留意されたい。

　また本章では，監査員が医薬品製造施設での品質システム，特にCAPA，リスク分析・管理を主眼に監査し，品質の高い，安全な医薬品を製造することに取り組んでいるかを，実際の手順，記録の検証を基に行えるようにまとめている。

1 Quality Management System／品質システム

基本の確認事項

本書のⅠ章で示したように，医薬品品質システムの基本的要件は原薬と製剤で大きな変わりはなく，有効性のあるシステムになっているかどうか，ICH Q10などで示される経営層の責務が規定されているかといった点が基盤となる。

チェック項目	チェック NO	Requirement／要求事項	Questions／監査時の質問例	PIC/S GMP Guide Part I NO.
Quality Assurance （品質保証）	Ⅱ-1	There must be a comprehensively designed and correctly implemented system of Quality Assurance incorporating Good Manufacturing Practice.	Are products designed and developed based on the requirements of GMP?	Principle
		GMPに即して，品質保証のシステムが適切に設計され整っていること	製品設計・開発は，GMPの要求事項を満たしていますか？	
	Ⅱ-2	Managerial responsibilities are clearly specified.	Dose the responsibility of management layer define under ICH Q10?	1.5, ICH Q10
		経営層の責任が明確化されていること	経営層の責任は，ICH Q10に基づいて明確化されていますか？	
	Ⅱ-3	Approved and documented self inspection schedule, which covers all GMP activities available.	Are internal audits being performed as scheduled? Can they be substituted by third party audits? How is the frequency of internal audits a year determined? Who has responsibility?	1.1, 9.Principle
		承認され，文書化されたGMPを網羅した自己点検のスケジュール	計画に則して，内部監査が行われていますか？ 内部監査は，第3者監査に代替できますか？ 内部監査の頻度は？ 内部監査の責任者は？	

1 Quality Management System

チェック項目	チェック NO	Requirement／要求事項	Questions／監査時の質問例	PIC/S GMP Guide Part I NO.
Product Quality Review (PQR)（製品品質照査）	Ⅱ-4	Regular PQRs performed in a timely manner (e.g. within three months from the end of the period being evaluated). Data from in-process controls, batch release analysis and other key quality indicators are included.	Is the data evaluated for the presence of trends, and are these acted upon? Are complaint, out-of-specification (OOS) and deviation investigations, reported, considered and evaluated in the PQRs? Are the PQR results used to revaluate the expected monitoring ranges in Batch Manufacturing Records?	1.10
		通常の品質照査は，定められた期間内に行われること（例：照査対象期間終了後，3カ月以内）。出荷，工程管理など重要な管理指標が含まれていること	品質照査にはトレンドを評価したデータは含まれていますか？ 苦情，OOS，逸脱調査は，品質照査に報告，考察，評価されていますか？ 品質照査は，製造記録の管理値（幅）の再評価に用いられますか？	
	Ⅱ-5	A review of OOS, critical IPC and API test results, deviations, complaints, returns and recalls, non-conformances and related investigations, including the effectiveness of the corrective and preventive actions conducted.	Are required changes highlighted in the PQRs implemented through the change control system?	1.10
		OOS，工程検査・原薬の品質試験結果の重要項目，苦情，逸脱，返品・回収，異常とそれらの調査とCAPAの有効性を照査すること	変更管理システムを経て準備された品質照査で，要求された変更は重要視されますか？	
	Ⅱ-6	Based upon the review, the validation status of a manufacturing process is evaluated and recorded.	Show me the example of PQR. Are there criteria for revalidation based on the review?	1.10
		この照査によって，製造工程のバリデーションの状況が評価・記録されること	年次照査の例を示してください。 照査に基づいて，再バリデーションを行う基準がありますか？	
Quality risk management（品質リスクマネジメント）	Ⅱ-7	ICH Q9 is introduced.	Is there quality risk management system in your facility? QRM procedure is documented?	1.13
		ICHQ9の導入	工場にリスク管理の手法がありますか？ リスク管理の手順は文書化されていますか？	

2 Personnel／従業員

生産を支えるに足る体制

人員が充足していることや，必要・十分な知識，資格を有する人材を確保していることが重要となる。重要な職責を担う従業員は，Key Personnelとして，他部門の責任者の併任禁止などが規定されている。

チェック項目	チェックNO	Requirement／要求事項	Questions／監査時の質問例	PIC/S GMP Guide Part I NO.
General（一般）	Ⅱ-8	There must be sufficient qualified personnel to carry out all the tasks which are the responsibility of the manufacturer.	Are there adequate numbers of personnel in facility? Is qualification of personnel sufficient at different levels in-place?	2.1
		十分に教育訓練を受け認証された人員数の確保	施設は十分数のスタッフが従事していますか？ 各部門で，認定された人材は充足していますか？	
	Ⅱ-9	Individual responsibilities should be clearly understood by the individuals and recorded.	Are responsibilities of all personnel engaged in manufacture in products is documented and available?	2.2
		個々の責任は個々のスタッフに認識され，記録されること	製造部門のすべての従業員の責任（職務）は文書化してありますか？	
Key Personnel（重要人員）	Ⅱ-10	The heads of Production and Quality Control must be independent from each other.	Are heads of Production and Quality Control independent from each other? Are there job definition, responsibility and organization chart?	2.5
		製造部門と品質部門の長は兼任できない	製造部門と品質部門の長は独立していますか？ 職務規定，組織図はありますか？	
Training（教育訓練）	Ⅱ-11	All personnel should be aware of the principles of Good Manufacturing Practice that affect them and receive initial and continuing training.	Is regular training conducted? Are records of training maintained?	2.10, 2.11
		すべての従業員（経営層・管理職を含む）は，GMPの原則を理解しており，初任者教育と継続教育を受けること	教育訓練は定期的に行われていますか？ 教育訓練記録は保管してありますか？	

チェック項目	チェック NO	Requirement／要求事項	Questions／監査時の質問例	PIC/S GMP Guide Part I NO.
Training（教育訓練）	Ⅱ-12	Visitors or untrained personnel should, preferably, not be taken into the production and Quality Control areas.	Do you have any training program/ orientation for Visitor/ Freshmen (including of Auditors)？ Untrained personnel are slickly prohibited to enter the Production and/or Quality control area?	2.11
		外部者，新人は，適切な教育訓練を受けなければ，製造区域・品質管理試験室には立ち入らせないこと	監査者を含め外部者，新人に対する教育訓練・導入プログラムが備わっていますか？ 教育訓練が終了していない作業員は，製造区域・品質管理試験室には立ち入ることが禁止されていますか？	
Personnel Hygiene（従業員の衛生管理）	Ⅱ-13	Every person entering the manufacturing areas and Quality Control areas should wear protective garments appropriate to the operations to be carried out.	Does Personnel wear clean clothing suitable for activity？ Are there Additional protective apparel where necessary (e.g. filling rooms)？	2.18
		製造区域・品質管理試験室に入室するすべての作業員は，作業に適した保護具を装着すること	従業員は業務に適した清潔な更衣をしていますか？ 必要な場合（例えば，充填室）は，追加の保護具を用いますか？	
	Ⅱ-14	Direct contact should be avoided between the operator's hands and the exposed product.	How is ensured that no direct contact with products, raw materials and intermediates？	2.20
		作業員が素手で露出した製品に接触することを防ぐこと	どのように，製品，原材料ならびに中間体に直接触れていないことを保証しますか？	
	Ⅱ-15	Rest room should be provided at isolated/ separated place from production/storage.	How is ensured that no smoking, drinking, chewing and storage of food takes place？	2.19
		休憩室は製造・保管区域より分離・隔離された場所に設ける	どのように，喫煙，飲食・チューインガム，食品の持込がないことを保証しますか？	
	Ⅱ-16	All operators in GMP are should be kept good health condition. Infection is not allowed to enter/contact.	How are personnel with infectious diseases identified？ Is there a procedure in place that these persons have no product contact？	2.17
		すべてのGMPに従事する従業員は，健康な状態にあること。感染者は，入場できない	どのように，感染者（罹病者）を識別しますか？ 感染者（罹病者）が，生産に携われないとの規定がありますか？	

3 Premises and Equipment／施設，機器

安定的製造に必要な事項

　施設，設備は，製品を製造するうえで十分なスペースが取られ，日常のメンテナンスの簡便性を考慮した設計になっていることが理想である。安定した品質の製剤を恒常的に造り続けるために必要なこと，という観点で監査を行うと，汚染防止や製品保管，混同防止などの対策が効果的なものか否かが見えてくる。

チェック項目	チェックNO	Requirement／要求事項	Questions／監査時の質問例	PIC/S GMP Guide Part I NO.
Premise-general（施設－一般）	Ⅱ-17	Premises should be situated in an environment which, when considered together with measures to protect the manufacture, presents minimal risk of causing contamination of materials or products.	Have procedures been implemented to protect the products and/or material from contamination through all stages of manufacture? (e.g. sieving, milling and packaging)	3.1
		構内は，製造を保護するための措置とともに，材料または製品の汚染を引き起こすリスクが最小限である環境に置かれることを考慮すること	手順は，すべての工程で，汚染から製品・原材料を守るように作られていますか？	
	Ⅱ-18	The level of product protection is dependent upon the product type and the expected time of exposure to the environment.	Have procedures been implemented to protect products and materials when exposed to each stage of the manufacturing environment?	3.1, 3.9
		製品の保護レベルは，製品の種別，環境に曝される時間に基づく	手順は，製造環境に曝されるとき，製品・原材料を守るように作られていますか？	
	Ⅱ-19	Premises and equipment must be located, designed, constructed, adapted and maintained to suit the operations to be carried out.	Have controls been implemented to ensure that the activities in surrounding areas/neighborhoods are not an actual source of contamination?	3.1, principle
		施設・機器は医薬品製造を行うに適するように，地区が選ばれ，設計・建設されねばならない	周囲の区域・隣接する活動が汚染の源にならないように管理・制御が確実になされていますか？	
	Ⅱ-20	Unauthorized personnel is not allowed to enter.	Are there any measurements to prevent the entry of unauthorized people? Production, storage and quality control areas?	3.5
		入場制限（承認された人員のみ入場可）	製造現場，保管場所，QC試験室へ許可されない人・物の入場を防ぐ手段がありますか？	
	Ⅱ-21	To prevent migration of pest animals.	Are facility designed and equipped to prevent against the entry of insects or other animals?	3.4
		害虫・獣の侵入防止	施設は害虫・害獣の進入を防止できるよう設計・設備をしていますか？	

3 Premises and Equipment

チェック項目	チェックNO	Requirement／要求事項	Questions／監査時の質問例	PIC/S GMP Guide Part I NO.
Premise-Production area（施設 – 製造区域）	Ⅱ-22	Production areas are strictly segmented/separation based on risk base.	Do you have measurement to ensure that highly sensitive products (penicillin and so on) and non-pharmaceutical materials (herbicides, pesticides, etc.) are not manufactured in the same building/equipment as used for Products.	3.6
		製造区域のリスクに応じた区分・分離	高感さ性の製品（ペニシリンなど）と非医薬品（除草剤，農薬など）が同じ建物／設備で製造されていないことを確認する方法がありますか？	
	Ⅱ-23	To minimize the risk of a serious medical hazard due to cross-contamination.	Are there dedicated and self-contained facilities available for the production of particular medicinal products, such as highly sensitizing materials (e.g. penicillin) or biological preparations (e.g. from live micro-organisms)?	3.6
		交叉汚染に起因する医学的危害のリスクを最小限にする	高感さ性物質（例えば，ペニシリン）または生物製剤（例えば，生きた微生物由来）のような，特定の医薬品の製造に利用可能な専用および独立型施設がありますか？	
	Ⅱ-24	The adequacy of the working and in-process storage space.	Does positioning of equipment and materials design to minimize the risk of confusion between different medicinal products or their components?	3.8
		製造区域，中間製品の保管庫は，十分な面積が必要	機器の設置場所，物資の保管場所は，混同のリスクを最小にするよう設計されていますか？	
	Ⅱ-25	Drain is big concerning on contamination from outside.	Are drains designed with adequate size, and to have trapped gullies? I necessary, do you order to facilitate cleaning and disinfection?	3.11
		排水路は，外部からの汚染の脅威である	排水口は十分な効力のある大きさと逆流防止を持つように設計されていますか？必要に応じて，製造所は施設の清掃・殺菌を依頼しますか？	
	Ⅱ-26	Weighing of starting materials usually should be carried out in a separate weighing room designed for such use.	Are weighing of starting materials usually carried out in a separate weighing room designed for dedicate purpose?	3.13
		出発材料の計量は，通常，そのために設計された独立の計量室で行う	出発物質の計量は，専用に分離した計量室で行いますか？	
	Ⅱ-27	Washing rooms might be source of cross contamination, and is required to keep good condition/cleanness.	Are washing areas appropriately managed and controlled? (equipment flow, storage of dirty and clean equipment, labeling)	3.37
		洗浄室は交叉汚染の原因になりやすいので，清潔な良好な状態に保たねばならない	洗浄区域は適切に管理されていますか？（作業の流れ，洗浄前・済みの保管，表示）	

第Ⅱ章 Audit Checklist for Finished Products／医薬品製剤製造所の監査チェックリスト

チェック項目	チェックNO	Requirement／要求事項	Questions／監査時の質問例	PIC/S GMP Guide Part I NO.
Premise-Storage Areas（施設—保管区域）	Ⅱ-28	Storage areas should be of sufficient capacity to allow orderly storage of the various categories of materials and products.	Does storage areas have sufficient capacity; space, function/facility to meet storage condition (temperature/humidity/sunlight) for storage of the various materials and products? e.g. starting and packaging materials, intermediate, bulk and finished products, products in quarantine, rejected, returned or recalled.	3.18
		多種多様の原材料・製品を整理整頓するために，保管場所は十分な容量・空間が必要	多種多様なものを保管するに適した条件（温度，湿度，遮光）に合致した機能・施設，面積，容積を持った保管区域がありますか？例えば，出発原料，包装資材，中間体，製品，さらに 検査中，不適合，返品・回収された製品など	
	Ⅱ-29	Condition of storage is key issue to prevent declining of materials quality.	Are storage areas designed or adapted to ensure good storage conditions? In particular, are they clean and dry and maintained within acceptable temperature criteria?	3.19
		保存条件は，製品の品質を劣化させないこと	保管区域は，良好な保管条件を保証できるように，設計されていますか？保管区域は，温度条件内に保たれ，清潔・乾燥状態に保たれていますか？	
	Ⅱ-30	Sampling room should be the function to prevent contamination.	If sampling is performed in the storage area, is it conducted to prevent contamination or cross-contamination?	3.22
		サンプリング室は，汚染防止の機能を持たねばならない	保管区域内でサンプリングを行うならば，交叉汚染防止を行っていますか？	
	Ⅱ-31	Special products are separately stored to prevent contamination/exposure.	Are highly active materials or products stored in safe and secure areas, separately?	3.24
		汚染・暴露を防止するため，特殊な物質は区分されること	高理活性（高感さ性）の原材料・製品は，分離して安全に保管していますか？	
	Ⅱ-32	Storage of label is required of security. (anti counterfeit).	Are printed packaging materials considered critical to the conformity of the medicinal products? Does special attention pay to the safe and secure storage of these materials?	3.25
		ラベルの保管はセキュリティの担保が求められる（偽薬防止）	印刷済み包装は，製品を区別するのに重要と考えられていますか？印刷済み包装の保管には，保安・安全に特別な注意がはらわれていますか？	

チェック項目	チェック NO	Requirement／要求事項	Questions／監査時の質問例	PIC/S GMP Guide Part I NO.
Premise-Storage Areas （施設－保管区域）	II-33	Storage status should be clearly defined to prevent mixed up.	Do you have well defined space/rooms for quarantine, approval and rejects material? Are there a restrict manner to control of access the defined raw materials? Are there systems to mark the status and ensure product security? Are there controlled rooms for retuned products and recalled products, and these rooms are clearly segregated?	3.21, 3.23
		保存のステータスは，混同を防止するよう，明確にされていること	製造所は，試験中，合格，不合格を明確に区別するに十分な広さを用意していますか？ 原料に接触できることは，厳格に管理されていますか？ 製品の保安管理・状況表示を行うシステムが整っていますか？ 返品・回収した製品の管理された部屋は準備されていますか？ その部屋は，隔離されていますか？	
Premise-Ancillary Areas （施設－付帯設備・施設）	II-34	Welfare of labor and to prevent contamination are required to be well organized.	Do you present rest and refreshment rooms that are separate from other areas?	3.30
		良好な作業者の福利厚生と汚染防止が十分になされていること	他の区域（製造）から離れた休憩室を提供できていますか？	
	II-35	Flow of human and location of Ancillary facility in the site are well designed.	Are facilities for changing clothes and for washing and toilet easily accessible and appropriate for the number of users?	3.31
		人の動線，福祉施設の位置は，適切に設計されること	更衣室，手洗い・トイレは，従業員数に見合っている数が準備され，容易に利用可能な状況にありますか？	
Equipment （機器）	II-36	URS of equipment should be well considered and clearly defined.	Are manufacturing equipment designed, located and maintained to meet its intended purpose	3.34
		ユーザー要求仕様書は，十分検討され，明確化されること	目的に合うように，すべての製造機器は設計，設置，管理していますか？	
	II-37	Maintenance and cleaning procedures of equipment are required "easiness" and clear description.	Are manufacturing equipment designed so that it can be easily and thoroughly cleaned? Are there cleaning procedures to be cleaned according to detailed and written procedures and stored only in a clean and dry condition?	3.36
		機器の保守点検，清掃の手順は，簡潔・明解な表現が求められる	製造機器は，簡単に，完璧に清掃できるように設計されていますか？ 文書化された清掃手順はありますか？ その文書には，清潔乾燥状態で保管することが明記されていますか？	

チェック項目	チェックNO	Requirement／要求事項	Questions／監査時の質問例	PIC/S GMP Guide Part I NO.
Equipment（機器）	Ⅱ-38	Measuring range might be suitable for purpose.	Do balances and measuring equipment have appropriate range and precision for production and control operations?	3.40
		測定範囲は目的に合っていること	秤・測定機器は，製造・管理のため適切な範囲・精度を備えていますか？	
	Ⅱ-39	Water should be distributed under clean condition.	Are distilled, deionized and other water pipes sanitized according to written procedures that detail the action limits for microbiological contamination?	3.43
		製造用水は，清潔な条件下供給されること	蒸留，脱イオン，その他の水質基準の水の管路は，微生物汚染限度（アクションレベル）が明記された手順に則して殺菌されますか？	
	Ⅱ-40	To avoid mixed up, clear labeling is required.	Are fixed pipework/equipment clearly labeled to indicate the contents and the direction of flow?	3.42
		混同防止のため，管路等に明解なラベルが求められる	設置された管路，機器は，内容物（生産中），使用の可否，流方向を明確に表示してありますか？	
	Ⅱ-41	Design and layout of equipment are to meet the intension of production, to prevent mixed-up/contamination.	Are Manufacturing equipment designed, located and maintained to suit its intended purpose? Show us the URS and DQ documents. Are Manufacturing equipment designed to be cleaned easily and thoroughly? Do you maintain equipment according to detailed and written procedures? Do you store manufacturing equipment after cleaning only in a clean and dry condition?	3.34, 3.36
		機器の設計・配置は，混同・汚染防止の意図に合致していること	すべての製造機器は目的に則して設計，設置，保守点検されていますか？ユーザー要求仕様書，DQの文書を提示してください。機器は，清掃が容易なように設計されていますか？機器は，詳しく文書化された手順に従って，保守されていますか？洗浄済みの機器は，清潔で乾燥状態に保管していますか？	

チェック項目	チェック NO	Requirement／要求事項	Questions／監査時の質問例	PIC/S GMP Guide Part I NO.
Equipment（機器）	II-42	Regular and preventive Maintenance is currently required to reduce risk.	Do you preventively repair and maintain equipment to avoid any hazard to the quality of the products? Are equipment installed to prevent any risk of error or of contamination? Show us the periodical maintenance plan and report with Quality review.	3.35, 3.38
		リスクを軽減するために，定期的・予防的保守点検が要求される	製造所は，製品の品質上の危害を防止するために，機器を予防的に保守点検しますか？ 設置された機器は，誤作動・汚染のリスクを防ぐことが行われていますか？ 定期的保守計画とその評価を見せてください	
	II-43	Balances and measuring is periodically calibrated to ensure quality assurance.	Are measuring, weighing, recording and control equipment calibrated and checked at defined intervals by appropriate methods? Are adequate records of such tests maintained?	3.40, 3.41
		品質の担保のため，定期的に秤，測定機器は校正が必要	測定機器，秤，記録機器，制御機器は，定められた間隔で，適切な方法で校正されていますか？ その校正記録は保存されていますか？	

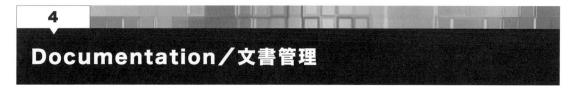

4 Documentation／文書管理

Good Documentation Practicesの考え方

文書管理の基本はGMPに共通するものだが，PIC/S GMP Guiceでは"Good Documentation Practices"の考え方が示されている点に留意して，監査を行う。各工程ごとに正確な記録が残され，文書化されていること，日付等に誤りがないことなど，データインテグリティの観点をもつことも重要である。

チェック項目	チェックNO	Requirement／要求事項	Questions／監査時の質問例	PIC/S GMP Guide Part I NO.
Generation and Control of Documentation（文書の生成と制御）	Ⅱ-44	Good documentation constitutes an essential part of the quality assurance system.	Written procedure in place describing preparation, review, approval and distribution of documents related to the manufacture?	4.1
		整備された文書は，品質保証システムの基幹の1つである	製造に関連する文書（手順）の準備，照査，承認，配布に関する文書は整っていますか？	
	Ⅱ-45	At site, the current/effective document is only in place.	How are revision, superseding and withdrawal of documents controlled?	4.5
		各現場では，有効な文書のみが備わっていること	どのように文書の改訂，配布，回収を行いますか？	
Good Documentation Practices（適正文書化規範）	Ⅱ-46	Any alteration made to the entry on a document should be signed and dated.	Is a revision history of SOP/standards/Specification maintained?	4.9
		文書に変更が加えられたならば，承認・署名（日時）がなされること	SOP，基準，規格の改訂履歴は残っていますか？	
	Ⅱ-47	Suitable controls should be implemented to ensure the accuracy, integrity, availability and legibility of documents. Instruction documents should be free from errors and available in writing.	Are corrected entries in documents dated and signed? Are there original entries still readable?	4.3, 4.9
		文書の正確性，一貫性，利用可能性，読みやすさを確実にするよう，適切な管理法が備わっていること。（製造）指示書は，誤謬がなく，記入可能なこと	文書中のすべての訂正は，日時と署名を記入してありますか？訂正前の内容を，読むことができますか？	

チェック項目	チェックNO	Requirement／要求事項	Questions／監査時の質問例	PIC/S GMP Guide Part I NO.
Retention of Documents（文書の保管）	Ⅱ-48	The raw data should be retained for a period at least as long as the records for all batches whose release has been supported on the basis of that validation exercise.	Do you define retention period for products with expiry date: 1 year after expiry (min.)? For investigational medicinal products, is the batch documentation kept for at least five years after the completion or formal discontinuation of the last clinical trial in which the batch was used?	4.11
		出荷されたすべてのバッチのすべての生データは，検証された期間（有効期限）は保管する	製造所は，記録の保管期間を最低有効期限＋1年間と定めていますか？治験に用いた製品では，当該の製品バッチが用いられた最後の治験が終了後もしくは中止後最低5年間は保管しますか？	
Specifications（規格）	Ⅱ-49	There should be appropriately authorized and dated specifications for starting and packaging materials, and finished products.	Are specifications for all raw materials, intermediates and products established?	4.13
		出発原料，包装資材，製品の規格書は適切に承認，日時が付記されていること	出発原料，中間体，製品の規格は制定されていますか？	
	Ⅱ-50	Specifications for intermediate and bulk products should be similar to specifications for starting materials or for finished products, as appropriate.	Are Specifications for intermediate and bulk products for critical steps documented?	4.15
		中間体・バルクの仕様は，必要に応じて，出発原料または完成品の仕様と同様でなければならない	重要工程に使用する中間体・バルク製品の規格は整っていますか？	
	Ⅱ-51	Specifications for finished products are key to disposition of any low quality and/or designed mater.	Does Specification contain the following items? -The designated name of the product and the code reference where applicable; -The formula; -A description of the pharmaceutical form and package details; -Directions for sampling and testing; -The qualitative and quantitative requirements, with the acceptance limits; --The storage conditions and any special handling precautions, where applicable; -The shelf-life.	4.16
		製品規格は，低品質または設計思想から外れた製品の出荷判断の要である	（製品）規格には次の項目が含まれていますか？・製品名・コード番号・構造式・医薬品としての定義，包装表示の詳細・サンプリングと試験の指示・適合基準（定性・定量）・保存条件，特別な注意事項・有効期限	

チェック項目	チェック NO	Requirement／要求事項	Questions／監査時の質問例	PIC/S GMP Guide Part I NO.
Manufacturing Formula and Processing Instructions - Packaging Instructions （製造指図 − 包装手順）	II -52	Requirement of items/format is defined in Guidelines to ensure proper packaging.	Does the Packaging instruction contain the following items? a) Name of the product; including the batch number of bulk and finished product; b) Description of its pharmaceutical form, and strength; c) The pack size expressed in terms of the number, weight or volume of the product in the final container; d) A complete list of all the packaging materials required, including quantities, sizes and types, with the code or reference number relating to the specifications of each packaging material; e) Where appropriate, an example or reproduction of the relevant printed packaging materials, and specimens indicating where to apply batch number references, and shelf life of the product; f) Checks that the equipment and work station are clear of previous products, documents or materials not required for the planned packaging operations (line clearance), and that equipment is clean and suitable for use; g) Special precautions to be observed, including a careful examination of the area and equipment in order to ascertain the line clearance before operations begin; h) A description of the packaging operation, including any significant subsidiary operations, and equipment to be used; i) Details of in-process controls with instructions for sampling and acceptance limits.	4.19

チェック項目	チェックNO	Requirement／要求事項	Questions／監査時の質問例	PIC/S GMP Guide Part I NO.
Manufacturing Formula and Processing Instructions - Packaging Instructions （製造指図－包装手順）		包装の要求事項・記録事項が定められている	包装指示書には次の項目が含まれていますか？ a) 製品名（バルク，製品のバッチ番号を含む） b) 医薬品の説明，力価 c) 最終包装形態には，製品の量・重量・数で表示された包装のサイズ d) 必要な包装資材の全リスト；それぞれの包装資材に関連して定められたコードをつけて，数量，大きさ，型 e) できれば，包装資材のサンプル／模型，ロット番号，有効期限の印刷位置指示見本 f) 製造場所・機器が，前の製品を除去しているか，包装計画に必要でない文書・機器がないか（ライン洗浄），機器が清浄・使用に適しているかのチェック g) 作業開始前に，ラインクリアランスを確認するため，場所・機器に細心の注意を払って調査することを含めての特別な注意事項 h) 使用される機器や重要な補助的作業を含む包装の記述（指示） i) サンプリングと規格の指示を含む工程検査の詳細	

チェック項目	チェック NO	Requirement／要求事項	Questions／監査時の質問例	PIC/S GMP Guide Part I NO.
Manufacturing Formula and Processing Instructions - Batch Processing Record （製造指図 ― バッチ記録）	II -53	Requirement of items/recording format is defined in Guidelines to ensure proper manufacturing and tractability.	Does the batch record contain the following items? a) The name and batch number of the product; b) Dates and times of commencement, of significant intermediate stages and of completion of production; c) Identification (initials) of the operator(s) who performed each significant step of the process and, where appropriate, the name of any person who checked these operations; d) The batch number and/or analytical control number as well as the quantities of each starting material actually weighed (including the batch number and amount of any recovered or reprocessed material added); e) Any relevant processing operation or event and major equipment used; f) A record of the in-process controls and the initials of the person(s) carrying them out, and the results obtained; g) The product yield obtained at different and pertinent stages of manufacture; h) Notes on special problems including details, with signed authorization for any deviation from the Manufacturing Formula and Processing Instructions; i) Approval by the person responsible for the processing operations. Note: Where a validated process is continuously monitored and controlled, then automatically generated reports may be limited to compliance summaries and exception / out-of-specification (OOS) data reports.	4.20

チェック項目	チェック NO	Requirement／要求事項	Questions／監査時の質問例	PIC/S GMP Guide Part I NO.
Manufacturing Formula and Processing Instructions - Batch Processing Record （製造指図 －バッチ記録）		製造の適格性とトレーサビリティを確実にするため，記録すべき条項・様式はガイドラインに定められている	製造記録には次の事項が含まれていますか？ a) 製品名・バッチ番号 b) 開始，重要な中間体の製造，製造終了の日時 c) 重要工程に従事した作業員の署名（イニシャル）と記録照査者名（必要に応じて） d) 実際に計量した原料とそのバッチ番号と試験番号（回収した原料，追加で添加した原料のバッチを含む） e) すべての関連する操作，出来事，主要製造機器 f) 工程試験結果とその試験を行った作業員のイニシャル g) 製品収量 h) 特別な問題の詳細を含む注記，"製造指示"からの逸脱に関する承認の署名 i) 工程責任者の照査と承認 注：バリデートされた工程を継続的にモニターする場合は，自動的に作成されのるは，遵守の要約，例外，OOSの報告に限られるかもしれない	
	Ⅱ-54	Batch Production Records are correct version. 記録が正しい版であること	Are Batch Production Records checked before issuance for correct version? 製造記録（指示書）は，事前に現在有効な版かを確認する手順になっていますか？	4.20
Procedures and Records – Receipt （手続きと記録 －受領）	Ⅱ-55	Receipt Records of Raw Materials, intermediates, product labeling and packaging materials is to ensure that manufacturing is started with the correct/qualified material.	Are Records of each delivery of raw materials containing? - name of manufacturer/supplier - identity and quantity - supplier control or identification number - number allocated on receipt - date of receipt - trace of use - review of labels and packaging materials showing conformity with specifications - final decision release or reject	4.23
		原材料，中間体，ラベル，包装資材の受領記録は，製造が正しい・認証したものを用いて製造開始した証拠となる	個々の原料の発送記録には次のことが含まれていますか？ ・製造者（供給者）の名称 ・原料の識別・量 ・供給者の管理（認証）番号 ・受領時の到着数量 ・受領日 ・密封性の確認（未使用，未開封の確認） ・外観：ラベル，容器外装（規格適合性） ・出荷判定	

チェック項目	チェックNO	Requirement／要求事項	Questions／監査時の質問例	PIC/S GMP Guide Part I NO.
Procedures and Records –Sampling（手続きと記録 — サンプリング）	Ⅱ-56	Requirement of items/format is defined in Guidelines.	Is procedure for sampling documented? Does the document include the methods and equipment to be used, the amounts to be taken and any precautions to be observed to avoid contamination?	4.25
		サンプリングの要求事項・記録事項は，ガイドラインに定められている	サンプリングの手順は文書化されていますか？ 文書には，(サンプリング）方法，用いる用具，採取する量，汚染防止のための注意事項が含まれていますか？	
Procedures and Records –Testing（手続きと記録 — 試験）	Ⅱ-57	Test is ensuring whether process is under going to respect standards procedure. And manufacturer will define the critical process/intermediate to demonstrate the constancy of procedures.	Do you define which samples on process will be investigated and documented all procedures? Show me the example of definition of sampling points and test results.	4.26
		試験は，工程が標準手順を遵守して行われているかの検証である。製造者は，工程・製造の安定性を証明するために，重要工程，中間体を定義する	全工程で，どの工程のサンプルを調査するか，文書化するかを決めていますか？ サンプル採取の箇所，その試験結果を見せてください	
Procedures and Records –other（手続きと記録 — その他）	Ⅱ-58	Lot number is required to identify the product and ensure tractability on manufacturing.	Are the records showing a unique batch number (not for continuous production)?	4.27, 4.28
		ロット番号には，製品を特定し，製造を追跡できることが求められる	特異的なロット番号をつけていますか？（連続生産を除いて，同一の番号は使用していませんか）	
	Ⅱ-59	Requirement of items/format is defined in Guidelines. Missing items is not allowed.	Are there records for the major equipment used , cleaning and maintenance showing the following - date - time - product and batch number of each batch - person who performed cleaning - person who performed maintenance	4.29
		記入項目・様式の要求項は，ガイドラインに決められている	重要な機器の使用，洗浄，保守記録はありますか？ 記録には，次の項目が含まれていますか？ 日時，製品名，バッチ番号，洗浄実施者，保守実施者	

Productions／製造

幅広く確認

混同や交叉汚染の防止といった，最終製剤の品質に直接的に影響が出る事項はもちろん，バリデーションや変更に関する点，包装資材に至るまで広く観察・監査する。

チェック項目	チェックNO	Requirement／要求事項	Questions／監査時の質問例	PIC/S GMP Guide Part I NO.
General（一般）	Ⅱ-60	Production operations must follow clearly defined procedures and record of procedure.	Does your document all procedure on receipt, quarantine, sampling labeling, dispensing of raw material and processing, packaging and distribution of products? Are all these handling procedures recorded, properly?	5.2
		製造操作は，明確に定義された手順と記録の手順に従う	受領，試験中，サンプリングラベル，原料の調合，製造，包装，製品の出荷などすべての手順を文書化していますか？すべての取り扱い手順は，適切に記録されていますか？	
	Ⅱ-61	To store all material to prevent adulteration, mixed-up or contamination.	Are all materials and products stored under the appropriate conditions to prevent contamination and quality decline?	5.7
		混同，品質低下，汚染防止をして，すべての原料を保管すること	すべての原材料，製品は，適切に品質の低下防止・汚染防止された条件下で保管されていますか？	
	Ⅱ-62	The measurement to prevent contamination and mixed up is required.	Do you operate process different products in the same room with the effective measurement to prevent risk of mix-up or cross-contamination?	5.9
		汚染・混同防止の手段が要求される	同一の生産区域で，混同，交叉汚染の効果的防止策を講じて，2種以上の異なる製品の製造を行いますか？	
	Ⅱ-63	To prevent cross contamination of foreign matter or biological infection.	Do you enforce to protect any stage of processing, products and materials from microbial and other contamination?	5.10
		微生物・異物等の混入を防ぐこと	微生物や他の汚染物から原材料・製品のあらゆる製造過程を守る努力をしていますか？	
	Ⅱ-64	The measurement to prevent Quality declining and to decrease impact to products is required.	Do you have appropriate storage system for materials, bulk containers, major items of equipment and labeling system to identify to prevent mixed up?	5.12
		品質の低下，製品への影響を低減する対策が要求される	適切な原材料，バルク製品，重要な生産機器の保管システム，混同防止のための識別ラベルシステムを持っていますか？	

チェック項目	チェックNO	Requirement／要求事項	Questions／監査時の質問例	PIC/S GMP Guide Part I NO.
Prevention of Cross-Contamination in Production（交叉汚染防止）	Ⅱ-65	The risk of accidental cross-contamination arises from the uncontrolled release of dust, gases, vapors, sprays or organisms from materials and products in process, from residues on equipment, and from operators' clothing.	Please show me the measurement to prevent Contamination of a starting material or a product by another material or product. Even from accidental source.	5.18
		工程中に原材料・製品，機器の表面に残る残渣，作業員の衣服から発生する管理できない塵埃，ガス，スプレー，微生物の偶発的な交叉汚染のリスクを防止する	出発物質の汚染防止，製品が他の製品からの汚染を防止する手順を示してください。偶然的な汚染源であってもです	
	Ⅱ-66	Cross-contamination should be avoided by appropriate technical or organizational measures.	Show me your policy and/or procedure to prevent Cross-contamination.	5.19
		適切な技術・組織的な手順で交叉汚染が防がれること	交叉汚染防止の手順・方針を示してください	
	Ⅱ-67	Efficiency to prevent cross contamination should be monitor.	Do you review the measures to prevent cross-contamination and their effectiveness periodically?	5.20
		交叉汚染防止の効果をモニターすること	定期的に交叉汚染防止の手順とその効果を照査しますか？	
Validation（バリデーション）	Ⅱ-68	To ensure the production procedure, validation is essential.	Do you conduct Validation studies under current guideline and document the validation procedures?	5.23
		製造の手順を確実にするため，バリデーションは必須である	最新のバリデーションのガイドラインに基づいてバリデーションを行い，手順を文書化していますか？	
	Ⅱ-69	Change control might give impact to quality, and is required of validation.	At change control of process and/or equipment, do you conduct Risk assessment management as Validation?	5.24, 5.25
		変更管理は品質に影響を与える可能性があり，バリデーションが必要である	工程，機器の変更時，バリデーションという手段でリスク評価を行いますか？	
	Ⅱ-70	Processes and procedures should revalidate periodically.	Do you conduct validation/revalidation for Processes and procedures based on risk based? After risk reduction procedure, do you conduct validation and/or confirm/evaluate the remaining Risk?	5.26
		工程，手順は定期的に再バリデーションされること	リスクベースで，手順・工程のバリデーション，再バリデーションを行いますか？ リスク低減の手順で，残存するリスクのためのバリデーション，確認・評価を行いますか？	

5 Productions

チェック項目	チェック NO	Requirement／要求事項	Questions／監査時の質問例	PIC/S GMP Guide Part I NO.
Starting Materials（出発物質）	II-71	Materials are qualified and evaluated to produce designed quality. 意図された製品を製造するため，原料は評価，認証されること	Do you purchase Starting materials from approved suppliers with defined specification? Show me the authorized Supplier list. 決められた規格，承認された供給業者から原料を購入していますか？ 承認された供給業者リストを提示してください	5.27
	II-72	Even different batches, each batch must be considered as separate for sampling, testing and release. バッチが異なれば，それぞれのバッチをサンプリング，試験して判定すること	Do you separately sample, test and release in the case one material delivery is made up of different batches? 同一原料で別のバッチ番号で入庫した場合，個別にサンプリング，試験，出荷判定をしますか？	5.31
	II-73	Appropriate procedures or measures to assure the identity of the contents of each container of starting material is required. 出発原料の個々の容器を検証する適切な手順・手段が必要	Do you conduct identity of the contents of each container of starting material? 出発物質は各容器（包装単位）に対して確認試験をしますか？	5.33
Processing Operation Intermediate and Bulk products（中間体，バルク製品の製造）	II-74	Quality of intermediate is kept under proper condition. 中間体の品質は，良好な条件に保たれること	Do you store Intermediate and bulk products under appropriate conditions with proper label to prevent contamination and quality decline? 中間体・バルク製品は，品質の低下・汚染を防ぐため，適切な表示を施し，最適な条件で保存されていますか？	5.41
	II-75	Before any processing operation is started, steps should be taken to ensure that the work area and equipment are clean and free from any starting materials, products, product residues or documents not required for the current operation. 作業を開始する前，作業エリアと機器が清潔で，作業に必要でない出発材料，製品，製品残留物，書類がないことを確認する	Before any processing operation is started, Do you ensure that the work area and equipment are clean and free of contaminate and/or remove all risk? 製造工程が開始する前には，製造区域・機器が正常である，コンタミがない，存在するリスクが除かれていることを確認していますか？	5.40

チェック項目	チェックNO	Requirement／要求事項	Questions／監査時の質問例	PIC/S GMP Guide Part I NO.
Packaging Materials（包装資材）	II-76	The selection, qualification, approval and maintenance of suppliers of primary and printed packaging materials shall be accorded attention similar to that given to starting materials.	Do you store printed material under secure condition? Are authorized personnel only allowed to access printed materials? Are the trailed label and/or loosed labels stored in the defined container to prevent mixed up? Do you record the release, attached, returned labels?	5.46
		一次包装および印刷包装材料の供給者の選択，資格認定，承認および維持は，出発材料に与えられたものと同様に注意を払わなければならない	印刷物は安全な条件で保管されていますか？ 印刷物にアクセスできるのは，許可された人に限られていますか？ 半端ラベル，開封したラベルは，混同防止のために別の容器に保管されていますか？ 出荷，添付，返却されたラベル（数）は記録していますか？	
Packaging Operation（包装工程）	II-77	The name and batch number of the product being handled should be displayed at each packaging station or line.	Do you indicate the name and batch number of the product in-operation at each packaging station or line to prevent mixed up?	5.51
		取り扱う製品の名称とバッチ番号を表示する必要がある	混同防止のために，包装区域・ラインには包装する製品名・バッチ番号を，表示していますか？	
Finished Products（最終製品）	II-78	Review of relative document on production and packing record is to ensure QMS and grantee the product quality.	Does Quality unit and release manager review all relative documents; batch record, quality test results, change/deviation control reports and approve before release of product? Show me the release certificate with Quality Unit approval.	5.63, 5.65
		製造・包装に関連する文書の照査は，製品の品質保証・QMSを担保する	品質部門・出荷判定責任者は関連するすべての記録を照査しますか？照査する文書：製造記録，品質検査結果，変更・逸脱管理報告と出荷前の承認 品質部門が承認した出荷判定書を見せてください	
Rejected, Recovered and Returned Materials（不適合，回収，返品物）	II-79	Clear labeling is key to prevent mixed up.	Do you attach reject label on the reject matter container and store at the defined/restricted room to prevent mixed up?	5.66
		正常なラベルは，混同防止の要である	不適合ラベルは不適合品容器に貼り付け，混同防止のために特定された場所に保管されていますか？	
	II-80	The reprocessing of rejected products should be exceptional.	As the conclusion of OOS, do you define the procedure of reprocessing as written procedure? Do you conduct risk assessment for reprocessing?	5.67
		再処理は例外でなければならない	OOSが判定されたとき，再処理の手順を定めていますか？ 再処理に関するリスク評価をしていますか？	

Quality Control／品質管理

業務規程

品質管理は試験室の運用に限定されるものではなく，製品品質に関係するあらゆる点に関与しなければならないという点が重要である．さらに品質部門は独立性を担保していることも必要で，幅広い業務を遂行するに足るだけの人員と経験を有することが求められる．

チェック項目	チェックNO	Requirement／要求事項	Questions／監査時の質問例	PIC/S GMP Guide Part I NO.
General（一般）	Ⅱ-81	Quality Control is not confined to laboratory operations, but must be involved in all decisions which may concern the quality of the product.	Is Quality control department independent from other departments? Is the authority of a person with appropriate qualifications and experience assigned?	6.1
		品質管理は実験室の運用に限定されるものではなく，製品の品質に関係するすべての決定に関与しなければならない	品質管理部門は他の部署から独立していますか？ 適切な資格と経験を持つ人の権限が割り当てられていますか？	
	Ⅱ-82	Enough number of Personnel is required.	Are there adequate resources available to ensure that all the Quality Control arrangements are effectively and reliably carried out?	6.1
		十分数の人材配置が要求される	品質管理を効率的に，現実的に行える十分数の人材が配置されていますか？	
	Ⅱ-83	To have job description of QC.	Does the Quality Control Department as a whole have duties, such as to establish? <example> - validate and implement all quality control procedures, - keep the reference samples of materials and products, - ensure the correct labeling of containers of materials and products, - ensure the monitoring of the stability of the products, - participate in the investigation of complaints related to the quality of the product, etc.	6.2
		品質管理の業務規定を有すること	品質検査部門は，次の例の業務の責任を持ちますか？ ・すべての試験法等の管理手順のバリデーションと遵守・履行 ・原材料・製品の参照品の保管 ・原材料・製品の容器／包装への添付ラベル管理・担保 ・製品の安定性の監視 ・品質に関する苦情の調査への参加	

チェック項目	チェックNO	Requirement／要求事項	Questions／監査時の質問例	PIC/S GMP Guide Part I NO.
Good Quality Control Laboratory Practice （適正品質管理室規範）	Ⅱ-84	Quality lab should have suitable facility, equipment to conduct quality control task.	Does Control Laboratory premises and equipment meet the general and specific requirements for Quality Control?	6.5
		品質管理業務を遂行するに適した施設・機器を備えていること	品質管理試験室は，品質管理に適した施設・機器を備えていますか？	
	Ⅱ-85	The personnel, premises, and equipment in the laboratories should be appropriate to the tasks imposed by the nature and the scale of the manufacturing operations.	Are the personnel, premises, and equipment in the laboratories qualified/prepared to meet to the tasks?	6.6
		従業員，施設および設備は，製造作業の性質および規模によって課される作業に適切であること	品質試験業務を行うに，試験室の人員，施設，機器は，適格性を検証されていますか？	
	Ⅱ-86	Segmentation of analysis room based on items.	Are there separate rooms to protect sensitive instruments from vibration, electrical interference, humidity, etc.?	3.28
		試験項目に則して，分析室は分割する	敏感な機器が振動，電気的妨害，湿度等から守られるように，部屋が分けられていますか？	
	Ⅱ-87	Special Quality control room for aseptic, high potential product and high sensitive product.	Are there special requirements in laboratories to hand particular substances, such as sterile, biological or sensitive samples?	3.29
		無菌，高活性物質，高感さ性製品用の特別品質管理室	取り扱いに特別に注意を要する製品（無菌，生物由来，感さ性）に関して特別な規定がありますか？	

チェック項目	チェック NO	Requirement／要求事項	Questions／監査時の質問例	PIC/S GMP Guide Part I NO.
Documentation（文書化）	Ⅱ-88	To have required documents on quality control procedure.	Are next Documents define and file to the Quality Control Department? - specifications; - sampling procedures; - testing procedures and records (including analytical worksheets and/or laboratory notebooks); - analytical reports and/or certificates; - data from environmental monitoring, where required; - validation records of test methods, where applicable; - procedures for and records of the calibration of instruments and maintenance of equipment.	6.7
		品質管理に要求される文書を有すること	次の文書が，品質管理部門で定義・保管されていますか？ ・規格書 ・サンプリング手順 ・試験法と記録様式（ワークシート，ラボノートを含む） ・試験報告，CoA ・環境モニタリングデータ（必要に応じて） ・試験法のバリデーション（該当する場合） ・試験機器の校正・保守点検の手順および記録	
	Ⅱ-89	Retention period of documents.	Do you retain any Quality Control documentation relating to a batch record for one year after the expiry date of the batch?	6.8
		適切な期間文書を保管すること	製造記録に関連する品質検査報告文書は有効期限＋1年以上保管しますか？	

チェック項目	チェックNO	Requirement／要求事項	Questions／監査時の質問例	PIC/S GMP Guide Part I NO.
Sampling（サンプリング）	Ⅱ-90	Requirement of items/procedure defined in Guidelines for sampling should be documented.	Do you have documented Procedure for sampling including the next articles? Do you respect Sampling procedure? - the method of sampling; - the equipment to be used; - the amount of the sample to be taken; - instructions for any required sub-division of the sample; - the type and condition of the sample container to be used; - the identification of containers sampled; - any special precautions to be observed, especially with regard to the sampling of sterile or noxious materials; - the storage conditions; - instructions for the cleaning and storage of sampling equipment. Show me the logbook for sampling of raw materials.	6.11
		サンプリングの要求事項・手順がガイドラインに定められている	次の項目はサンプリングの手順に含まれていますか？ この手順を遵守していますか？ ・サンプリングの方法 ・サンプリングに使用する器具 ・採取するサンプル量 ・（採取した）サンプルの分割法 ・採取したサンプルの容器タイプと状態 ・容器の識別法 ・無菌・有害物への特別な注意事項 ・保管条件 ・サンプリングに使用する器具の洗浄・保管法 サンプリングのログブックを提示してください	
	Ⅱ-91	Sampling container is kept to be clean and identified to prevent contamination and mixed up.	Are sample containers appropriately labeled and kept clean to avoid mixed-up and contamination?	6.13
		サンプリングに用いる容器は，汚染防止・混同防止のために，清潔・識別がなされていること	サンプル容器は，汚染防止・混同防止のために，識別がなされ，清潔に保たれていますか？	

チェック項目	チェック NO	Requirement／要求事項	Questions／監査時の質問例	PIC/S GMP Guide Part I NO.
Sampling（サンプリング）	II-92	Reference (retain) sample is retained to demonstrate quality of the product and ensure tractability on manufacturing.	Do you have the program/procedure to keep Reference samples from each batch of finished products for one year after the expiry date? Are retained finished products kept in their final packaging and stored under the recommended conditions?	Annex 19-3.1
		参照（保持）サンプルは，製品の品質を実証し，製造上の取り扱いやすさを保証するために保持されること	それぞれの生産バッチから参考品をとり，有効期限＋1年間保管するプログラム・手順がありますか？ 参考品は，最終包装形態で，推奨される保存条件で保管されていますか？	
Testing（試験）	II-93	Implementation of analysis Method validation.	Are analytical methods validated?	6.15
		分析法バリデーション	分析法はバリデートされていますか？	
	II-94	Requirement of items/format is defined in Guidelines.	Do you record of test procedure and their results? Are there the data included the following items? a) name of the material or product and, where applicable, dosage form; b) batch number and, where appropriate, the manufacturer and/or supplier; c) references to the relevant specifications and testing procedures; d) test results, including observations and calculations, and reference to any certificates of analysis; e) dates of testing; f) initials of the persons who performed the testing; g) initials of the persons who verified the testing and the calculations, where appropriate; h) a clear statement of release or rejection (or other status decision) and the dated signature of the designated responsible person. i) Reference to equipment used.	6.17
		試験法の要求事項・手順が定められている	試験手順とその結果は記録していますか？ 試験記録には，次の項目が含まれていますか？ a) 試験物質，製品名（剤形） b) バッチ／ロット番号（製造業者名） c) 品質規格・試験法 d) 試験結果，観察事項・結論とCoAに引用される項目 e) 試験日 f) 試験実施者 g) 試験記録のチェック者，再計算者 h) 判定（出荷許可，不適合）と承認責任者の署名，日時 i) 使用機器のリファレンス	

チェック項目	チェック NO	Requirement／要求事項	Questions／監査時の質問例	PIC/S GMP Guide Part I NO.
Testing（試験）	Ⅱ-95	In-process controls should be performed according to methods approved by Quality Control and the results recorded.	Who will take sample for in-process? Do you define the sampling procedures and document? Does Quality unit approve the procedure and documents?	6.18
		工程管理試験は，QCで承認された手法で行われ，記録されること	工程試験のサンプルは誰が採取しますか？ サンプリングの手順は規定され，文書化されていますか？ 品質部門は手順を承認していますか？	
	Ⅱ-96	Laboratory reagents should be marked with the preparation date and the signature of the person who prepared them. The expiry date of unstable/common reagents and culture media should be indicated on the label with specific storage conditions.	Do you have the labeling system for lab reagents and inventory lists of reagent? Do you define the expiry date of reagents/solution/medium based on Scientific evidence?	6.21
		試験室の試薬，調整液は，調整者の署名，調整日を表示すること。通常試薬・安定でない試薬・培地の使用期限は，保存条件をラベルに表示すること	試薬のラベルシステムと在庫リストが整っていますか？ 試薬・調整液・培地の有効期限は科学的な根拠に基づいていますか？	
On-going Stability Program（年次保存安定性）	Ⅱ-97	The purpose of the on-going stability program is to monitor the product over its shelf life and to determine that the product remains.	Do you have the enough stability data to support own shelf-life/expiry date? Do you have the monitoring program to demonstrate stability that the product remains?	6.27
		年次の保存安定性試験は，使用期限を確かめ（確認），製品の有効性が残存していることを目的とする	有効期限を担保する十分な保存安定性試験結果を保持していますか？ 有効期間内製品がその特性・性能を保持していること担保するモニタリングプログラムを持っていますか？	
	Ⅱ-98	After marketing, the stability of the medicinal product should be monitored according to appropriate program.	Do you have post marketing stability program for any products? Do you annually review the stability program?	6.26
		上市後，適正なプログラムに従って，製品の安定性をモニターしなければならない	すべての製品が，市販後安定性試験プログラムの対象ですか？ 年次で，安定性試験プログラムを見直しますか？	

チェック項目	チェック NO	Requirement／要求事項	Questions／監査時の質問例	PIC/S GMP Guide Part I NO.
On-going Stability Program （年次保存安定性）	II-99	The protocol for an on-going stability programme should extend to the end of the shelf life period.	Do you have the protocol for on-going stability program to extend expiry date/shelf-life? What kind of parameter Do you will evaluate? Are there the Protocols containing the following parameters as minimums? Does the protocol for an on-going stability program to extend to the end of the shelf life period include? - number of batch(es) per strength and different batch sizes, if applicable - relevant physical, chemical, microbiological and biological test methods - acceptance criteria - reference to test methods - description of the container closure system(s) - testing intervals (time points) - description of the conditions of storage (standardized ICH conditions for long term testing, consistent with the product labeling, should be used) - other applicable parameters specific to the medicinal product.	6.30
		プロトコールは，保存期間の終わりまで延長する必要があり，必要なパラメータが定められている	使用期限を延長するための保存安定性試験プロトコールを持っていますか？ どのようなパラメータを保存安定性で定めていますか？ 次の項目を安定性試験プロトコールに含んでいますか？ ・使用するバッチ番号・力価 ・関連する物理化学的，微生物学的分析法 ・合格基準（規格値） ・参照分析方法 ・容器仕様 ・試験間隔 ・保存条件（ICH基準，ラベル記述の保存条件） ・その他；特殊なパラメータ	
	II-100	The number of batches and frequency of testing should provide a sufficient amount of data to allow for trend analysis.	Do you adapt for annual stability program with at least one batch per year of product manufactured in every strength and every primary packaging type? Do you define the frequency of testing based on risk-based approach?	6.32
		バッチの数とテストの頻度は，傾向分析を可能にするのに十分な量のデータを提供する必要がある	すべての力価，1次包装単位で最低年1バッチについて年次保存安定性試験を行っていますか？ リスクベースアプローチに基づいて試験の頻度を決めていますか？	

チェック項目	チェックNO	Requirement／要求事項	Questions／監査時の質問例	PIC/S GMP Guide Part I NO.
Technical transfer of testing methods （試験法技術移転）	Ⅱ-101	The parameters that should be included in transfer protocol is defined.	Do you have the protocol for Technical transfer of testing methods? Are there included the following items? (i) Identification of the testing to be performed and the relevant test method(s) undergoing transfer; (ii) Identification of the additional training requirements; (iii) Identification of standards and samples to be tested; (iv) Identification of any special transport and storage conditions of test items; (v) The acceptance criteria which should be based upon the current validation study of the methodology and with respect to ICH/VICH requirements.	6.39
		試験法移転プロトコールに含まれる事項が定められている	試験法技術移転のためのプロトコールはありますか？ 次の項目が含まれていますか？ (i) 実施される試験の識別および移転される関連試験方法 (ii) 追加の訓練要件の特定 (iii) 試験される基準および試料の特定 (iv) 試験項目の移転および保管条件の特定 (v) ICH／VICH要件に基づいた直近のバリデーションによる合格基準	

Outsourced Activities／委託

委受託関係での連携

委託者，受託者ともに求められる要件があるが，いずれにしても品質契約に基づいて連携が図られていることが必要である。技術移転については労力がかかる部分であるので，本書では簡単な確認チェックリストを示しているが，詳細は他の専門書等も参考にしていただきたい。

チェック項目	チェックNO	Requirement／要求事項	Questions／監査時の質問例	PIC/S GMP Guide Part I NO.
General（一般）	Ⅱ-102	There should be a written contract covering the outsourced activities, the products or operations to which they are related, and any technical arrangements made in connection with it.	Did the firm enter the Quality agreement with contractor before technical transfer would be started?	7.1
		書面による契約と定義があること	技術移転の開始前に，品質契約が締結されていますか？	
The Contract Giver（委託者）	Ⅱ-103	Technical transfer between contract giver and acceptor.	Has firm accomplished technical transfers between you and contractor under international guidance? Are the technical transfer processes documented and the reports reviewed/approved by Quality Unit?	7.4
		委託主と受託先の間での技術移転	国際的ガイダンスに基づき，技術移転がなされましたか？ 技術移転は文書化され，品質部門の照査・承認を得ていますか？	
The Contract Acceptor（受託者）	Ⅱ-104	Capability and comprehensive on technical of contractor.	Is your contractor a reliable partner on view points; adequate premises/equipment, knowledge and experience, and competent personnel?	7.6
		受託者の能力と技術理解度があること	充足した施設・機器，知識と経験，能力ある人材という観点から，委託先は信頼できる相手ですか？	
	Ⅱ-105	Sub-contractor is defined under Quality agreement.	Does your contactor assign the sub-contractor on analysis and/or manufacturing under the original quality agreement? Do you recognize the situation of Sub contractor and controlling by the contractor?	7.8
		品質契約には，再委託について規定すること	品質契約の下に，再委託製造・分析が規定されていますか？ 委託先が再委託先の管理状況，再委託先の状況を認識していますか？	

チェック項目	チェック NO	Requirement／要求事項	Questions／監査時の質問例	PIC/S GMP Guide Part I NO.
The Contract (契約)	Ⅱ-106	In the agreement, responsibility process and control items should be defined.	Are there quality agreement between your Firm and contractor to specify their respective responsibilities relating to the manufacture and control of the product?	7.11
		品質契約に，責任体制・管理項目が規定されること	製品の製造・管理に関する責任体制を定めた，2社間の品質契約が取り交わしてありますか？	
	Ⅱ-107	Audit to contract manufacturer.	Does Contractor agree to audit the facilities by Product owner and/or third parties?	7.14
		委託製造先監査	受託者は，委託者・第3者による監査実施を認めていますか？	

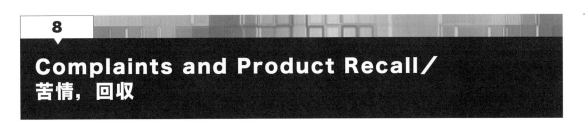

Complaints and Product Recall/苦情,回収

迅速な対応を

苦情,回収はPIC/S GMP Guideの中でも重要視される。回収に関わる事項は速やかに当局に情報を伝達することが必要で,その手順がしっかりと定められていることが重要である。また,重大な問題の場合は,患者リスクを考え,迅速に回収を行える体制が整っていることも確認すべきである。

チェック項目	チェックNO	Requirement/要求事項	Questions/監査時の質問例	PIC/S GMP Guide Part I NO.
Personnel and Organisation（人員と組織）	Ⅱ-108	A person should be designated responsible for handling the complaints.	Who is the compliant manager? To whom, does compliant manager report the significant compliant?	8.1
		苦情処理の責任者を任命すること	誰が苦情責任者ですか？ 重大な苦情に関して誰に報告しますか？	
Procedures for Handling and Investigating complaints including possible quality defects（品質問題を含む苦情の取り扱いおよび調査）	Ⅱ-109	There should be written procedures describing the action to be taken, including a recall.	Do you have documented procedure on compliant? Are there procedures of communication to authorities and to consider recall in the case of critical hazardous?	8.5
		回収を含め,苦情の対応の手順が文書化されていること	苦情対応の手順がありますか？ 重大な苦情の場合,当局への連絡や回収を検討する手順が整っていますか？	
	Ⅱ-110	Firm has the responsively to investigate impact of compliant and/or possibility of product failure in other lots.	Do you have the system that all the decisions and measures taken as a result of a complaint are recorded and referenced to the corresponding batch records?	8.10, 8.11
		苦情の影響,他のロットで不適合（不都合）がないかの調査の責任を有す	すべての苦情の対応に基づき取られた結果・対応手段を記録,関連する製造記録を照査するというシステムを持っていますか？	
Root cause analysis and Corrective and Preventive Action（原因分析と是正／予防措置）	Ⅱ-111	As compliant handling, CAPA is essential procedures and indication of CAPA is required.	Do you have the CAPA procedure to significant complaints?	8.18
		苦情処理には,CAPAの手順が必要,CAPAの指示も求められる	重要（重篤）な苦情に対してCAPAの手順を適用させますか？	

チェック項目	チェックNO	Requirement／要求事項	Questions／監査時の質問例	PIC/S GMP Guide Part I NO.
Root cause analysis and Corrective and Preventive Action （原因分析と是正／予防措置）	II-112	Complaint records and reports are evaluated in the PQRs in order to identify trends, product related frequencies, and severity.	Are complaints correctly evaluated in PQRs? (i.e. is there any evaluation of reoccurrence and trends?) Are corrective/preventive actions managed through the change control system?	8.19
		苦情記録および報告は，トレンド，頻度，重篤度を特定するためにPQRで評価されること	苦情は，年次照査で評価されますか？（再発，トレンドの評価結果はありますか？） （苦情に伴う）変更管理にて，CAPAは管理されますか？	
Product Recalls and Other potential risk-reducing actions （回収とリスク低減活動）	II-113	Recall procedure must be documented.	Do you manage all complaints properly? Are the record and results properly recorded?	8.20
		手順は文書化が必須	すべての苦情を適切に取り扱っていますか？ 苦情の受領，対応結果は適切に記録していますか？	
	II-114	All concerned Competent Authorities should be informed in advance in cases where products are intended to be recalled. For very serious issues, rapid risk-reducing actions (such as a product recall) may have to be taken in advance of notifying the Competent Authorities.	Show me the notification address list on recall. Is there a procedure to recall quickly for serious problems?	8.25, 8.26
		関係するすべての管轄当局は，製品が回収される予定は事前通知を受けるべき。深刻な問題については，管轄当局に通知する前に，迅速なリスク低減行動（製品回収など）を行う必要がある	連絡一覧表を見せてください。 深刻な問題の場合には，迅速に回収を行う手順になっていますか？	

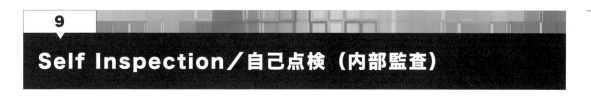

Self Inspection／自己点検（内部監査）

効果のある自己点検か

定期的に自己点検を行って，しっかりと記録が残されているかを確認する。ただ形だけ行う自己点検で中身が伴っていないということがないか，GMPに定められている項目をしっかりと押さえているかを確認する目が必要になる。

チェック項目	チェックNO	Requirement／要求事項	Questions／監査時の質問例	PIC/S GMP Guide Part I NO.
Principle（原則）	II-115	Item on self inspection is defined in PIC/S GMP guide.	Do you conduct self-inspection, periodically? Are there items of Self-inspections including of next items? - Personnel matters, (Job, training etc.) - premises, - equipment, - documentation, - production, - quality control, - distribution of the medicinal products, - arrangements for dealing with complaints and recalls, - self-inspection (follow)	9.1
		自己点検の項目は，PIC/SのGMPガイドに従う	定期的に，自己点検を行いますか？ 自己点検には，次の項目が含まれていますか？ ・人員（分担，教育訓練） ・施設 ・機器 ・文書 ・製造 ・品質管理 ・流通 ・苦情処理，回収 ・自己点検（前回のフォロー）	
	II-116	To assign auditor for self-inspection has no interest relationship.	Do you assign the self-inspection auditors as independent and qualified personnel? Do you have the training program for Self-inspections?	9.2
		内部監査員は，該当部署とは利害関係がないこと	内部監査（自己点検）者は，利害関係がなく，認定された人材を指名しますか？ 自己点検のための教育訓練プログラムがありますか？	

チェック項目	チェックNO	Requirement／要求事項	Questions／監査時の質問例	PIC/S GMP Guide Part I NO.
Principle （原則）	Ⅱ-117	All self inspections should be recorded.	Do you record all self-inspections? Do reports contain all the observations made during the inspections and, where applicable, proposals for corrective measures?	9.3
		すべての自己点検は記録されること	すべての自己点検の報告書がありますか？ すべての報告書には内部監査で発見された指摘事項が含まれていますか？好ましくはCAPAが含まれていますか？	

10 Manufacture of Liquids, Creams and Ointments／液剤，クリーム，軟膏の製造

ここでは，PIC/S GMP Annex 9の内容を基に監査のチェックリストを提示する。液剤，クリーム剤特有の要件も存在するため，ANNEX 9の要件を踏まえたうえで，以下チェックリストを適宜アレンジして使用されたい。

チェック項目	チェックNO	Requirement／要求事項	Questions／監査時の質問例	PIC/S GMP Guide Annex 9 NO.
Premises and equipment（施設および設備）	Ⅱ-118	Closed systems of processing and transfer is recommended. 閉鎖系システムが推奨される	Is production areas where the products or open clean containers are exposed normally effectively ventilated with filtered air? 製品，洗浄後の未封容器が環境に曝される製造区域は，効果的に浄化された空気で覆われていますか？	1
Production（製造）	Ⅱ-119	The chemical and microbiological quality of water used in production should be specified and monitored. 水の化学的および微生物学的品質を特定し，監視すること	Is "Care of chemical and microbiological quality of water" taken in the maintenance of water systems in order to avoid the risk of microbial proliferation? 微生物の増殖のリスクを避けるため，「水質の化学的および微生物的品質の管理」は行われていますか？	4
	Ⅱ-120	Care should be taken to maintain the homogeneity of mixtures, suspensions, etc. during filling. 充填中の混合物，懸濁液などの均質性を維持するように注意する必要がある	Is special care taken at the beginning of a filling process, after stoppages and at the end of the process to ensure that homogeneity is maintained? 製品の均一性を担保するため，製造開始，中断後，製造終了時に，特別な充填工程管理が行われますか？	8
	Ⅱ-121	When the finished product is not immediately packaged, the maximum period of storage and the storage conditions should be specified and respected. 最終製品が直ちに包装されない場合は，最大保管期間および保管条件を指定すること	Are the maximum period of storage and the storage conditions specified and respected? 最長の保存期間，保存条件は定義され，遵守されていますか？	9

11 Manufacture of Biological Medicinal Substances and Products for Human use／ヒト用生物学的医薬原薬および製剤の製造

　ここでは，PIC/S GMP Annex 2を基本としながら，その他要件も含めて，生物由来製品に関する監査の簡単なチェックリストを提示する。製品によって細かな要件も多いため，交叉汚染防止等，基本的な内容についてのチェックリストをまとめた。必要に応じて，確認項目を追加してほしい。

チェック項目	チェックNO	Requirement／要求事項	Questions／監査時の質問例	PIC/S GMP Guide Annex 2 NO.
Personnel（従業員）	Ⅱ-122	Prevention of cross contamination.	Please show me your procedure to avoid the simultaneous handling of other living or infectious material by the same persons! Do workers pass to other areas during one working day? Show me your Log books	4
		交叉汚染防止	同じ人が他の生体物または感染性のある物質を同時に取り扱うことを防ぐ手続きを示してください 作業者は就業日中，他の作業区域を通過することはありますか？ ログブックを見せてください	
	Ⅱ-123	Procedure to avoid the simultaneous handling of inactivated products and active ones by the same persons should be in place.	Do workers pass from areas with active products to inactivated products (general) areas?	4
		同一作業者が，活性状態の製品（物）と不活性化したものを同時に扱うことを防ぐ手順が備わっていること	作業者は，（微生物）活性がある製品を取り扱っている区域から不活性化された製品を扱う（一般的な）区域に行くことがありますか？	
	Ⅱ-124	To have the concept of hygiene.	Do you have a concept of hygiene including change of clothes, masks, gloves, disinfection? Do you have emergency procedure under particular circumstances?	3
		衛生管理方針をもつこと	衣服，マスク，手袋，消毒剤の交換など，衛生に関する基本方針はありますか？ 特定の状況下での緊急手順を有していますか？	

11 Manufacture of Biological Medicinal Substances and Products for Human use

チェック項目	チェックNO	Requirement／要求事項	Questions／監査時の質問例	PIC/S GMP Guide Annex 2 NO.
Premises（施設）	Ⅱ-125	To keep the facility and environmental to meet Manufacturing. Equipment and environmental particulate and microbial contamination should be controlled.	Do you classify the room/area to the activities, appropriately? Do you design the rooms and equipment appropriate to the activities? How do you define the pressure difference (positive, negative, sink, containment)? Do you have negative pressure areas or safety cabinets used for aseptic processing of pathogens surrounded by a positive pressure sterile zone? Do you have the rooms product dedicated? Do your HVAC systems work adequate? How to demonstrate? Do you have a separation concept of areas and rooms to avoid cross contamination for the whole company? Do you have a concept of environmental monitoring? Do you monitor the pressures and/or pressure difference? Do you have Procedure to operate fumigation? Do you have any procedures and a management in case of missing of integrity and damage? Do you have a system to break dedicated area?	6
		施設・機器は製造に適した状態に維持する。特に環境機器は，交叉汚染を防止するよう管理すること	活性がある製品を取り扱っている区域／部屋を適切に分類していますか？ 活性がある製品に適するように部屋や設備を設計していますか？ 差圧（正，負，低下傾向，封じ込め）をどのように定義しますか？ 陽圧滅菌ゾーンに囲まれた病原体の無菌処理をする負圧区域または安全キャビネットはありますか？ 微生物）活性がある製品専用の部屋がありますか？ HVACシステムは適切に機能していますか？どのように証明するのですか？ 会社全体で，交叉汚染防止のための区域・部屋の分離の方針を持っていますか？ 環境モニタリングの方針はありますか？ 圧力や圧力差を監視していますか？ 燻蒸(殺菌)を行う手順がありますか？ 完全性の欠如と損害が生じた場合の手順，管理手順はありますか？ 専用エリアを開放するシステムがありますか？	

11 ヒト用生物学的医薬原薬および製剤の製造

チェック項目	チェックNO	Requirement／要求事項	Questions／監査時の質問例	PIC/S GMP Guide Annex 2 NO.
Equipment（機器）	Ⅱ-126	To prevent contamination of inactivated products by activated ones.	Do you use the same equipment used both for decontamination and sterilization? Please indicate flows of contaminated materials and equipment separated from those of sterilized ones. Do you validate effluents decontaminations inter-campaign and periodically revalidate?	8, Part Ⅱ -18.15
		微生物活性製品からの非活性製品への汚染防止	同じ機器を除染と滅菌の両方に使用していますか？ 滅菌済みのものから分離した汚染された材料や装置の流れを示してください。 キャンペーン間の排水汚染を検証し，定期的に再検証しますか？	
Starting Materials（出発物質）	Ⅱ-127	To keep defined Storage conditions.	Do you define and document storage conditions for all intermediates and drug substance and drug product?	36 Part Ⅱ -18.2
		保存条件を適切に維持	すべての中間体，原薬および医薬品の保管条件を定義し文書化していますか？	
Operating Principles（運用原則）	Ⅱ-128	Critical operational (process) parameters, or other input parameters which affect product quality, need to be identified, validated, documented and be shown to be maintained within requirements.	Do you define and document all process parameters (e.g. pH, temperature, time, flow rate)?	Part Ⅱ -18.13, 18.14
		重要な操作（プロセス）パラメータ，または製品品質に影響する他の入力パラメータは，識別され，検証され，文書化され，要件内で維持されること	すべてのプロセスパラメータ（例えば，pH，温度，時間，流量）を規定し，文書化していますか？	
Waste Material（廃棄物の廃棄）	Ⅱ-129	To inactivate waste material.	Do you validate the method to disinfect waste material?	Part A-59
		廃棄物は不活化すること	廃棄物を不活性化する方法をバリデートしていますか？	

チェック項目	チェックNO	Requirement／要求事項	Questions／監査時の質問例	PIC/S GMP Guide Annex 2 NO.
Bio technological Drug product （バイオテクノロジー医薬品）	Ⅱ-130	To confirm that it meets the standard.	Do you have the procedure to confirm/test products to meet Specification? Please indicate the specification and test procedures following; • Quality; physical & chemical properties (e.g. appearance, particulates, pH, moisture ...) • Identity • Protein concentration • Content Purity/Contamination (viral, pyrogens, microbial, chemical) • Activity (potency) • Sterility	Part Ⅱ -18.14
		規格を満たすことを確認	規格項を満たすことを確認，または/テストする手順はありますか？ 以下の規格とテスト手順を明記してください ・品質，物理・化学的性質（外観，粒度，pH，水分など） ・確認試験 ・タンパク質含量 ・含量，純度・不純物（ウイルス，微生物，有機・無機不純物） ・力価 ・無菌性	

第 III 章

Audit Checklist for Plant/Laboratory Tour／プラント／ラボツアー実施のためのチェックリスト

　監査時，必ず行うプラント／サイトツアーを想定して，製造設備・施設，一般品質試験室ならびに微生物試験室に立ち入り，実物の製造設備機器・品質試験機器等を前にして，担当者に尋ねる，確認すべき項目を具体的なチェックリスト・質問例として準備した。「百聞は一見に如かず」のことわざに従い，製造現場ならびに品質試験・微生物試験室において，監査員が直接作業員，担当者（分析者）に尋ねることを想定して，基本的な質問をまとめた。

　単に施設内を見学するのでなく，GMPの概念を含め，その製造所が，堅牢な品質システムを維持，改善しているか，その証拠となる文書が出せるかを目的としている。

1 Plant Tour／プラントツアー

効率的な確認を

プラントツアーでは，効率的に文書システムや設備の概要，汚染防止策が取られているかなどを確認する。

チェック項目	チェック NO	Requirement／要求事項	Questions／監査時の質問例	PIC/S GMP Guide NO.
APIs specific areas / activities（原薬の特定区域・活動）	Ⅲ-1	If bulk deliveries are made in non-dedicated tankers, there should be assurance of no cross-contamination from the tanker. バルク原材料が非専用タンクに運び込まれる場合，タンクからの交叉汚染防止を確実にすること	Are the general condition of tanks and ancillary equipment (pumps, pipes, vents, etc.) appropriate for their intended use? Are all tanks and associated pipes appropriately labeled and secure? タンクと付随設備（ポンプ，管路，バルブなど）は使用目的に合致するよう全般の状態は適切に保全されていますか？ タンクと管路は適切に表示・保全されていますか？	Part Ⅱ-7.22
	Ⅲ-2	Cleaning procedures should contain sufficient details to enable operators to clean each type of equipment in a reproducible and effective manner. 洗浄手順は，作業員が装置を再現性よく効果的に洗浄するための十分な詳細さで記載されていること	Are washing areas appropriately managed and controlled? (equipment flow, storage of dirty and clean equipment, labeling) 洗浄区域は適切に運用・管理されていますか？ （機器の流れ，洗浄前・済みの機器の保管，表示）	Part Ⅱ-5.21
Air conditional system（空調システム）	Ⅲ-3	Adequate ventilation, air filtration and exhaust systems should be provided, where appropriate. 適切な場所に，適切な換気，空気ろ過および排気システムを提供すること	Does the HVAC system provide an appropriate environment for finishing areas where APIs are exposed? 原薬が暴露される最終的な区域にHVACシステムは適切な環境（空気清浄度）を担保しますか？	Part Ⅱ-4.21, 4.22
Key design parameters（設計時の要件）	Ⅲ-4	To design to prevent/minimize Cross contamination.	How do you prevent cross contamination by air? Are there design on following items? Need for separate systems - Level of filtration (Filter specifications) - Recirculation or makeup air - Location of filters - Position of inlet and air return, dust extractors - Temperature Humidity - Air changes - Pressure differentials - Design of ducting - Easy and effective cleaning - Alarm system - Air flow direction- LAF and/or turbulent	Annex 1-27

チェック項目	チェックNO	Requirement/ 要求事項	Questions/ 監査時の質問例	PIC/S GMP Guide NO.
Key design parameters（設計時の要件）		交叉汚染防止もしくは最小限にするよう設計すること	製造所はどのように汚染防止を行っていますか？ 設計（仕様）には次の項目を含んでいますか？ ・フィルターのグレード（フィルターの仕様） ・清浄空気は循環するか ・フィルターの設置場所 ・吸気，循環気流，塵埃除去の位置 ・温度・湿度 ・換気回数 ・差圧 ・排気の方式 ・洗浄のしやすさ，有効性 ・警報システム ・噴出した気流の方向性，整流と乱流	
Qualification of HVAC Systems（HVACシステムの適格性評価）	Ⅲ-5	Qualification of HVAC systems should be completed.	How have you implemented recommendations and correct deviations mentioned in qualification reports? Qualification reports have the next items? • DQ, IQ, OQ and PQ • Average speed and uniformity of airflow • Pressure differentials • Air changes • Integrity and tightness of terminal installed final filters Who is responsible for evaluating if requalification is necessary?	Annex 1-68
		HVACシステムの適格性確認テストを行うこと	適格性報告書に記述されている逸脱の是正と推奨はどのように実施されましたか？ 項目には以下が含まれていますか？ ・DQ/IQ/OQ/PQ ・気流速と気流の均一性 ・差圧 ・換気回数 ・最終フィルターの完全性 再適格性評価が必要なとき，誰が責任者ですか？	

チェック項目	チェックNO	Requirement/要求事項	Questions/監査時の質問例	PIC/S GMP Guide NO.
Qualification of HVAC Systems（HVACシステムの適格性評価）	III-6	To confirm confront differences between design specifications, drawings (in SMF) and reality, unplanned maintenance and change control.	How do you challenge your alarm systems? Place and procedure for sampling? Where and how do you weigh and refill starting materials? Are rooms for the production of medicinal products equipped with HVAC in accordance with GMP requirements1? • Location of filters • Position of inlets and air return • Dust extractors, • Pressure differences (across filters, between production and adjacent rooms) • Logbooks-maintenance and calibration • Monitoring of other process parameters • HVAC alarm systems function	Annex 1-68
		SMFに記述の仕様と実際の使用に差がないか，計画にない保守・変更管理がないかを確認する	アラームシステムのチャレンジ試験はどのように行いますか？ 製造所はどこで，どのように出発物質を計量・仕込みますか？ 医薬品製造現場には，GMPの要求項に則したHVACが設備されていますか？ ・フィルターの位置 ・空気の噴出しと戻りの位置 ・塵埃除去器の設置 ・差圧（フィルターの前後，製造室と隣接の部屋） ・保守点検・校正記録 ・他の工程モニター項目 ・HVACの警報機能	
Monitoring of HVAC Systems（HVACシステムのモニター）	III-7	To monitor necessary items.	Is there including the following items? • Environmental monitoring (particles, micro organ, humidity, temperature • Chemical residue testing • Integrity test for HEPA filter with PAO	Part II-4.22
		必用な項目をモニタリングしていること	（モニタリングには）次の項目が含まれていますか？ ・環境モニタリング（浮遊微粒子，微生物，湿度・温度） ・化学物質残留試験 ・HEPAフィルターの完全性試験	
Maintenance and Calibration of HVAC Systems（HVACシステムの保守点検・校正）	III-8	Maintenance / calibration items are appropriate.	The interaction between unplanned maintenance and requalification is required. Is there including the following items? - Maintenance program - Calibration program - SOP - Records - Breakdown/Emergency including challenges of alarm systems	Part II-4.20

1 Plant Tour

チェック項目	チェックNO	Requirement/要求事項	Questions/監査時の質問例	PIC/S GMP Guide NO.
Maintenance and Calibration of HVAC Systems（HVACシステムの保守点検・校正）		保守・点検の項目が適切であること	予定外の保守・変更と再適格性の間での相互影響評価は，下記の点を含んでいますか？ ・保守点検計画 ・校正計画 ・手順書（SOP） ・記録書 ・アラームシステムのチャレンジ試験を含む，緊急・停止時の対応	
Documentation for HVAC Systems（HVACシステムの文書）	Ⅲ-9	Required items are documented.	Are there documentation on following items? • Technical data • SOP, records; maintenance, calibration, validation, monitoring, deviations, change control • Validation protocols and reports • As–built engine drawing	Part Ⅱ-12.2, Annex 15
		必要なことが文書化されていること	下記の項目に関して文書化されていますか？ ・技術的データ ・手順書，記録（保守点検・校正・バリデーション・モニタリング・逸脱・変更管理） ・バリデーションの計画と報告書 ・完成図面	
Water（水）	Ⅲ-10	The tap water is acceptable to suitable for intended use.	Are records of CoA available? Has testing at an appropriate frequency been conducted? Does potable water meet at the minimum WHO guidelines? (e.g. free from chemicals such as carcinogens, toxic substances, heavy metals, organochlorine pesticides, lindane, DDT, organic compounds, etc.; radiological and microorganisms)	Part Ⅱ-4.30, 4.31, 4.32 WHO Guidelines for drinking-water quality
		水道水は使用目的に合致した規格であること	CoAの記録は閲覧可能ですか？ 妥当な間隔で水源を評価していますか？ 水道水は，最低限WHOの基準を満たしていますか？ （有機物，有機塩素系残留農薬（DDT, リンデンなど），有機化合物，放射性物質，微生物などを含まないこと）	
	Ⅲ-11	The warter treatment process should be validated and monitored with appropriate action limits.	If water treated by the manufacturer, has the treatment process been validated? Have the effects of seasonal variation and human activity on the water quality been addressed? Is the process monitored?	Part Ⅱ-4.33
		水処理の工程はバリデーションすること。適切なアクション基準に基づき監視すること	水処理法は検証されていますか？ 生活排水や四季変動を考慮していますか？ プロセスは監視されていますか？	

チェック項目	チェックNO	Requirement/要求事項	Questions/監査時の質問例	PIC/S GMP Guide NO.
Water （水）	III-12	Water used in the final isolation and purification steps should be monitored and controlled.	Is the water used in the final isolation and purification steps monitored and controlled for microbial counts, objectionable organisms and endotoxins?	Part II - 4.34
		最終的な分離・精製に使用される水は，モニター，管理すること	最終的な分離・精製に使用される水は，微生物限度，対象生物やエンドトキシンをモニター，管理していますか？	
Water quality grade （水質）	III-13	Water quality grade and purposes of its use.	How is the system kept in a validated state? Let me have a look in the sight glass. Show me the records of alarms that have occurred. Is water for injection produced and used according to requirements of Note for Guidance on Quality of Water for Pharmaceutical Purposes? Are there any differences between drawings and reality, unplanned maintenance and change control? Follow the system from pre-treatment to user points: in each part, check leaks, sampling points (access), who does what, start up and shutdown?	Part II - 4.33
		水処理システムの品質確認	どのように，最適な状態に維持していますか？　内部を見せてください。 警報が発せられた（試験）記録を見せてください。 注射用水は，水質に関するガイダンスの製造法に則していますか？ 図面と実際の配管に差がありますか？ 不作為の保守・変更がありますか？ 前処理からユースポイントをたどって，漏れは検査していますか，サンプリングポイントは誰がどのように開放して，採取して，閉じますか？	
Monitoring of Warter （水のモニタリング）	III-14	Where to find responsibility for monitoring and corrective action.	By whom and how are corrective actions made? For example, you found any indication as over limit: - Temperature - Speed - Vent filters - DI column regeneration - pH - UV light (PW) - Conductivity - Leakage - TOC	Part II - 4.32 Annex 1-59

チェック項目	チェックNO	Requirement/要求事項	Questions/監査時の質問例	PIC/S GMP Guide NO.
Monitoring of Warter（水のモニタリング）		是正措置とモニタリングの責任の所在	誰がどのように，水質の是正措置を行いますか？例えば，下記の項目で，異常値が検出されたとき： ・温度 ・水流速 ・ベントフィルター ・イオン交換樹脂カラムの再生 ・pH ・紫外線殺菌（精製水） ・導電率 ・水漏れ ・TOC	
Maintenance and calibration of Water Systems（水システムの保守点検と校正）	Ⅲ-15	The maintenance plan is documented and implemented.	The interaction between unplanned maintenance and requalification is confirmed? - Maintenance program - Calibration program - SOPs - Records - Breakdown/Emergency including challenges of alarm systems	PartⅠ-3.41
		保守計画が文書化され実施されていること	予定外の保守・変更と再適格性の間での相互影響評価は，下記の点を含んでいますか？ ・保守点検計画 ・校正計画 ・手順書（SOP） ・記録書 ・アラームシステムのチャレンジ試験を含む，緊急・停止時の対応	
Documentation of Water Systems（水システムの文書化）	Ⅲ-16	All records, reports and procedures are documented.	Are there documentation on following items; - Drawing – up to date (Site Master File is current version?) - OOS evaluation - Deviation reports - Change control reports - Operation of the system - Cleaning / sanitation /sterilization - Logbook – monitoring parameters- see 1.6, incidents, filter changes, shut down periods, cleaning/sanitation, maintenance	PartⅠ-4, PartⅡ-6
		すべての記録，報告書，手順が文書化されていること	これらは文書化されていますか？ ・管路図面（SMFの最新版） ・OOSの評価（調査結果） ・逸脱報告書 ・変更管理報告書 ・システムの運転手順 ・洗浄，殺菌記録 ・ログブック：管理指標のモニター，フィルター交換，機器の始動，閉鎖，洗浄・滅菌，保守点検	

チェック項目	チェックNO	Requirement/要求事項	Questions/監査時の質問例	PIC/S GMP Guide NO.
Flow of materials and personnel (動線)	Ⅲ-17	Flow of material and personnel are appropriate for process.	Show me the Flow of material and personnel. Are the flow of materials and personnel appropriate for the processes? Are appropriate indications displayed in critical areas? (Gowning instructions, labeling for clean/unclean areas, incoming/out-coming materials, etc.)	Part Ⅱ-4.13
		人と物の動線がプロセスに通じていること	人と物の動線を示してください。この動線、工程上適していますか？動線図には、重要な区域に適切な指示書が示してありますか？例：更衣室での更衣手順、洗浄室の洗浄前・済みの表示方法、受入れ物と排出物の指示、	
Containment (封じ込め)	Ⅲ-18	Design of the multipurpose use containment area.	Has the containment area been qualified for multipurpose use?	Part Ⅱ-4.4
		封じ込め区域を多品種製造に設計	封じ込め区域は、多品目生産用に評価されていますか？	
	Ⅲ-19	If air is recirculated to production areas, appropriate measures should be taken to control risks of contamination and cross-contamination.	If HVAC is not dedicated, what controls are in place to prevent cross-contamination?	Part Ⅱ-4.22
		空気を生産地域に再循環させる場合は、汚染や相互汚染のリスクを管理するための適切な措置を講じること	HVACが専用でない場合、どのような交叉汚染を防ぐ管理が準備されていますか？	
Design (設計)	Ⅲ-20	Defined areas or other control system for different activities (Storage, sampling, quarantine, production, etc.).	Are there any definition on segmentation between GMP facility and non-GMP facility?	Part Ⅱ-4.10, 5.10
		区域の定義、もしくは他の活動の管理システム（保管、サンプル採取、試験中、製造など）	GMP適用施設と非GMP適用施設の間の分離は定義がありますか？	
	Ⅲ-21	Potential contamination and cross contamination has been prevented by the location and placement of equipment.	Is there policy to prevent contamination?	Part Ⅱ-4.10
		区域、機器の設置場所により潜在的な汚染や交叉汚染を防ぐ	汚染防止の方針・規定はありますか？	
Pharmaceutical Steam Systems, Key Design Parameters (蒸気システムの基本設計)	Ⅲ-22	Appropriate items should be considered at design time.	Are there design on following items? • entrainment prevention • no cross-contamination • clean steam • non condensable • gases reduction • slope of pipe-works • no dead legs	Part Ⅱ-4.10, Annex 15-8.1

1 Plant Tour

チェック項目	チェックNO	Requirement/ 要求事項	Questions/ 監査時の質問例	PIC/S GMP Guide NO.
Pharmaceutical Steam Systems, Key Design Parameters（蒸気システムの基本設計）		設計時に適切な項目が考慮されるべき	次の項目を考慮して、設計されていますか？ ・巻き込み防止 ・交叉汚染防止 ・清浄蒸気 ・凝縮水なし ・ガスを除去 ・適切な管の勾配 ・滞留箇所なし	
Pharmaceutical Gases, Key Design Criteria (compressed air)（圧縮空気ガスの設計基準）	Ⅲ-23	Appropriate items should be considered at design time.	Are there design on following items? • air inlet-source, contamination risks • filters (pre – final) • suitability of materials • welding • prevention of contamination (receiver vessel) valves	Part Ⅱ- 4.20, Annex 15- 9-10
		設計時に適切な項目が考慮されるべき	設計には下記の項目が含まれていますか？ ・吸入口（汚染のリスク） ・フィルター（プレ，最終） ・適正材料 ・溶接技術 ・汚染防止機能バルブ	
Qualification of Utilities（ユーティリティの適格性評価）	Ⅲ-24	All utilities that could impact on product quality (e.g. steam, gases, compressed air, and heating, ventilation and air conditioning) should be qualified and appropriately monitored.	How do you assure utilities? How do you define that filters are replaced in time? How do you conduct DQ, IQ, OQ, PQ? How do you prevent contamination of solid contaminants, water, oil limits? How do you define capacity, filter pressure drops, alarm operation?	Part Ⅱ- 4.20～23, Annex 15
		製品の品質に影響を及ぼす可能性があるすべてのユーティリティ（蒸気，ガス，圧縮空気，暖房，換気，空調など）は，適格であり，適切に監視されていること	どのようにユーティリティの適正を保証しますか？ フィルターが適正に交換されるようにどのように定めますか？ DQ，IQ，OQ，PQはどのように運営しますか？ 固形，水，油などの異物混入をどのように防ぎますか？ 能力，圧損，使用警告をどのように決めますか？	

チェック項目	チェック NO	Requirement/要求事項	Questions/監査時の質問例	PIC/S GMP Guide NO.
Identify all used gases with the risk for medicinal products （使用しているガスの製品へのリスク）	Ⅲ-25	Confirm the differences between drawings and reality, unplanned maintenance and change control.	Note Review item on walk through; - contact with the product or with the "process equipment" - type of the product (terminally sterilized, aseptic procedures) - labeling and identification of the system - risk of mix up - Identify all other used gases	Part Ⅱ - 5.11, 4.34
		図面と実際の管路の差異，不作為の保守・変更を確認	観察ポイント ・製品または製造機器との接触 ・製品種類（最終滅菌，工程滅菌） ・表示，システムの認識 ・混同に直結するリスク ・使用目的が異なるガス	
Operating Systems （運転システム）	Ⅲ-26	Maintenance of filter.	Note Review item on walk through; ・Changing system for filters ・SIP system ・Back-up systems ・Capacity-consumption	Part Ⅱ - 4.20, 4.21, 6.20
		フィルターの保守	観察ポイント ・フィルターの交換 ・殺菌・滅菌システム ・バックアップシステム ・ガスの供給量・消費量	
Quality Control （品質管理）	Ⅲ-27	Prevention of contamination of equipment and equipment.	Note Review item on walk through ・Pollution - oil ・water ・particles ・bioburden	Part Ⅰ - 3.43, 6.7
		機器および装置の汚染防止	観察ポイント ・機械油の混入：ミスト ・水分 ・微粒子 ・バイオバーデン	
Maintenance and Calibration of the Systems （保守・校正）	Ⅲ-28	Prevention of deterioration of equipment and equipment.	Are there the interaction between unplanned maintenance and requalification confirmed? ・Maintenance program ・Calibration program ・SOP ・Records ・Breakdown/Emergency including challenges of alarm systems	Part Ⅰ - 3.41
		機器および装置の劣化防止	予定外の保守・変更を確認していますか？ ・保守点検計画 ・年次校正計画 ・SOP ・記録 ・アラームシステム（チャレンジ試験を含む）	

チェック項目	チェックNO	Requirement/ 要求事項	Questions/ 監査時の質問例	PIC/S GMP Guide NO.
Documentation of utilities (ユーティリティの文書化)	Ⅲ-29	Drawings for these utility systems should be available.	Note Review item on document review; • Line drawings (pipeline, flow, valves, filters, rooms) • Deviation and corrective actions • Cleaning / sanitation / sterilization • Logbook – monitoring parameters, incidents, filter changes, shut down periods, cleaning /sanitation, maintenance	Part Ⅱ - 4.20
		ユーティリティの図面を備えること	観察ポイント ・管路図；フィルター，流路，バルブ，配置 ・逸脱・変更管理 ・洗浄・殺菌 ・ログブック；モニターする項目，異常，フィルター交換，管路閉鎖（不使用）期間，洗浄・殺菌，保守記録	

2 Lab Tour in Chemical and Physical-Chemical Laboratories／化学および物理化学ラボでのラボツアー

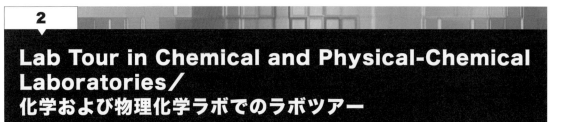

確認項目を順に点検

製造区域同様，ラボにおいても，確認すべき事項をあらかじめ洗い出しておき，効率的かつ網羅的に質問するように心がけることが必要である。

チェック項目	チェックNO	Requirement／要求事項	Questions／監査時の質問例	PIC/S GMP Guide NO.
Premises（施設）	Ⅲ-30	Location of the QC laboratories Facility design, rooms separation (e.g. clean and dirty, different testing activities) should be considered including of temperature, humidity, ventilation and recording systems/alarms.	Are QC labs separated from production areas? Where type of testing is carried out e.g. chemical, biological (microbiological) testing? Is the laboratory equipment located in appropriate area (e.g. clean equipment in clean room)? How is the system of ventilation/humidification/temperature designed? Is it monitored continuously? Is this system separated for QC area from other areas? System of alarms for critical equipment exists? How are the documents/sensitive instruments protected? Are storage conditions monitored? Where is defective equipment stored? Is there clearly indicated of rooms, areas (directions), status? Are dedicated rooms/laboratories clearly identified?	Part Ⅱ-11, Part Ⅰ-6.5

チェック項目	チェック NO	Requirement/要求事項	Questions／監査時の質問例	PIC/S GMP Guide NO.
Premises (施設)		QCラボの適切な配置，施設設計，部屋の分離を行うこと（例えば，清潔が要求項，異なる試験項目）	QCラボは生産区域から分離されていますか？ 実施される試験のタイプは化学的，生物学的（微生物学的）試験ですか？ 実験室の設備は適切な場所に設置されていますか（クリーンルームにクリーン度測定機器など）？ 換気／湿度／空調システムはどのように設計されていますか？ 継続的に監視されていますか？ QCエリアの換気／湿度／空調システムは他のエリアから分離されていますか？ 重要な機器のアラームシステムは存在しますか？ 文書／機密文書はどのように保護されていますか？ 保管状態は監視されていますか？ 不良品はどこに保管されていますか？ 部屋，エリア（道順），状態表示が明確に示されていますか？ 専用の試験室は明確に識別されていますか？	

チェック項目	チェックNO	Requirement/要求事項	Questions／監査時の質問例	PIC/S GMP Guide NO.
Equipment（機器）	Ⅲ-31	Documents necessary for the equipment to be used are maintained.	Do you have instructions for brief description of major equipment available? Relevant validation documents, SOP(s) for line with qualified assembly and documentation of all possible configurations available? Appropriate environmental conditions clearly stated? Is the Calibration procedure defined in the document? Documentation (e.g. records) available? Intervals for calibration defined? Calibration status indicated? Equipment status indicated? Exist for every major equipment? Are data complete? SOP(s) exists? Records available (require for critical equipment (as applicable))?	Annex 15-3
		使用機器には，必要な書類が整備されていること	主要機器の使用説明書はありますか？ 適格性に関連する妥当性確認文書，適格な組立ラインのSOP，使用可能なすべての構成の文書化がなされていますか？ 適切な環境条件が明確に示されていますか？ 校正手続きは文書で定義されていますか？ 文書（レコードなど）はありますか？ 校正の間隔は定義されていますか？ キャリブレーションの状態は？ 機器の状態が示されていますか？ 主要機器はすべて存在しますか？ データの完全性は保証されていますか？ SOPは存在しますか？ 使用記録（重要な機器）（該当する場合）がありますか？	

2 Lab Tour in Chemical and Physical-Chemical Laboratories

チェック項目	チェックNO	Requirement/要求事項	Questions／監査時の質問例	PIC/S GMP Guide NO.
Equipment（機器）	Ⅲ-32	Qualification is properly done.	IQ, OQ, PQ was carried out prior to first use? Who approves? Fully documented (including possible involvement of suppliers and/or third party)? Included intervals for revalidation? Requirements and specification for delivered equipment (URS) exists? Relevant checks were made? Details on specifications and acceptance criteria are provided? Operators have been trained? Sufficient details of procedures, materials and certified reference materials are available? Results are recorded in a manner amenable to establishing trends? Results are checked and evaluated by supervisor or delegate? Raw data are consistent with data in summary report? Results are within acceptance criteria applied?	Annex 15 - 3.2～3.14
		適格性評価が適切に行われていること	IQ, OQ, PQは最初に使用する前に実施しましたか？ 誰が承認するのですか？ 完全に文書化（サプライヤーおよび/または第三者を含む）されていますか？ 再適格性確認の間隔が含まれていますか？ 納入された機器の要件と仕様（URS）は存在しますか？ 関連するチェックが行われましたか？ 規格と受入れ基準の詳細事項は提供されていますか？ オペレーターは訓練を受けていますか？ 手順，材料および認定された標準物質の詳細情報は十分ですか？ 結果は，トレンドを把握するのに適した方法で記録されていますか？ 結果は監督者または代理人によってチェックおよび評価されますか？ 生データはサマリーレポートのデータと一致していますか？ 適格性確認テストの結果は受入れ基準内で適用されますか？	

チェック項目	チェックNO	Requirement/要求事項	Questions／監査時の質問例	PIC/S GMP Guide NO.
Cleaning, Sanitation（洗浄，衛生）	Ⅲ-33	Cleaning / sanitation system must be maintained.	Validation was carried out? Relevant documents available? What are the limits for equipment cleaning? Which equipment, glassware and other containers are used for cleaning/ sanitation? Who cleans? Is he/she trained? What are the intervals for cleaning areas specified? SOP is available?	Annex 15-10
		洗浄，衛生システムが整っていること	バリデーションは行われましたか？ 関連文書はありますか？ 機器の洗浄の制限はありますか？ 洗浄／衛生管理にどの機器，ガラス製品，その他の容器を使用していますか？ 誰が洗浄しますか？訓練を受けましたか？ 特定された洗浄すべき範囲の洗浄間隔はどのくらいですか？ SOPは利用可能ですか？	

チェック項目	チェック NO	Requirement/要求事項	Questions/監査時の質問例	PIC/S GMP Guide NO.
Maintenance（保守管理）	Ⅲ-34	Have a maintenance plan and document it.	How is maintenance programmed, performed and documented? Are the critical systems, areas, equipment included? Which work is contracted? Are the regular/extraordinary maintenance programs available? Who "releases" equipment after maintenance/repair for laboratory performance? Is there a schedule including time frames available? Is there inventory of items to be included into the maintenance system? Is there system for the formal acceptance of equipment back into service (and vice versa)?	Part Ⅱ - 4.20, 5.20, 6.60, 6.61
		保守管理計画を有し，文書化していること	メンテナンスはどのように計画され，実行され，文書化されますか？ 重要なシステム，エリア，機器はこの計画に含まれていますか？ どのメンテナンス作業が契約されていますか？ 定期的／特別なメンテナンスプログラムはありますか？ ラボの作業のためにメンテナンス／修理後に機器を承認する人はいますか？ 時間枠を含む利用可能なスケジュールはありますか？ メンテナンスシステムに含まれる項目の機器のリストはありますか？ 機器を正式に受け入れるシステムがありますか（逆も同様）。	

第Ⅲ章　Audit Checklist for Plant/Laboratory Tour／プラント／ラボツアー実施のためのチェックリスト

チェック項目	チェックNO	Requirement/要求事項	Questions／監査時の質問例	PIC/S GMP Guide NO.
Material Management (物質管理)	Ⅲ-35	Procedures for handling reagents, standards, toxic substances, hazardous substances, and sensitizing materials are provided, and they are properly operated.	List(s) of materials/reagents are available? The suppliers are listed, and are they assessed? What are requirements of identification tests? How is labelling (e.g. date of receipt)? Testing kits used? How new lots are traced back to the previous lots? How are Reference substances handled, labelled, stored (expiration)? Primary standards are available? Are the secondary Reference substances are acceptable? Traceability to official standards assessed? Working standards prepared? How used? Is there an SOP for the in-house calibration of reference materials? How expiry date and potency value are assigned to each reference standard/material characterized in–house? How are these reference standard/material handled (stored)? Are there relevant instructions available? Which measures are introduced to avoid cross contamination? Is SOP for waste disposal available?	Part Ⅱ - 11.16, 11.17

チェック項目	チェックNO	Requirement/要求事項	Questions／監査時の質問例	PIC/S GMP Guide NO.
Material Management（物質管理）		試薬，標準物質，毒性物質，有害物質，感さ性物質の取り扱い手順が規定されており，適切に運用されること	材料/試薬の一覧はありますか？ サプライヤーはリスト化され，評価されていますか？ 確認試験の要件は何ですか？ 材料/試薬のラベリングはどのように行われますか？（受領日など） テストキットが使用されていますか？ 新しいロットは以前のロットにどのように紐づけされますか？ 標準物質はどのように取り扱われ，ラベルが付けられ，保存されますか？ 基準はありますか？ 作業標準物質は許容されますか？ 正式な標準品へのトレーサビリティは評価されていますか？ 作業標準品は準備されていますか？どのように使用しますか？ 標準物質の社内校正のためのSOPはありますか？ 社内で認定された各標準品/材料に有効期限と校正値がどのように割り当てられていますか？ これらの参照標準品/材料はどのように取り扱われますか？ 関連する指示がありますか？ 交叉汚染を防止するためにどのような対策が採用されていますか？ 廃棄物処分のSOPはありますか？	

チェック項目	チェックNO	Requirement/要求事項	Questions/監査時の質問例	PIC/S GMP Guide NO.
Water and Water Systems（水，水システム）	III-36	To have a test water production system, quality standards, sampling and quality testing.	Is the laboratory water system described? How is the laboratory water prepared? Water quality is defined? Your specification on water are respecting Pharmacopoeia? What is the quality of water used for microbiological testing? Where, when and how is your laboratory water sampled (SOP)? What kind of quality testing is done for your water used for different types of analyses?	Part II-4.3
		試験水の製造システムがあり，品質規格，サンプリング，品質試験が正しく行われること	品質試験用の水システムは文書化されていますか？品質試験用の水はどのように供給されていますか？品質試験用水質は規格化されていますか？水に関する規格は薬局方に準拠していますか？微生物検査に使用される水の品質は？どこで，いつ，どのように品質試験用の水サンプルを採取しますか（SOPに定められていますか）？さまざまな品質試験の分析に使用される水について，どのような品質試験が行われますか？	
Sampling（サンプリング）	III-37	General policy of Sampling, Place of sampling for raw materials, Starting/packaging materials sampling, IPC's sampling /Intermediates sampling, System of air sampling, Procedures/records, Retained samples, Re-sampling aredefined.	Show me the description of sampling system (authorization, statistics application, sampling tools/areas). What is the number of samples taken and justification for reduced sampling? How is Sampling performed? By whom? Is SOP(s) for sampling available? Dose SOP include the details on containers, labelling, equipment cleaning etc.? Is there separate sampling area or area? How is the risk of cross contamination/bacterial contamination prevented? System of IPC's/intermediates sampling described (SOP)? What type of air sampler is used and why? What is the sample volume/testing time, media used, transfer time (SOPs)? Is equipment calibrated (have a protocol)? What disinfection procedure is used? What sampling techniques including equipment used? Show me the store for retained samples of raw materials and final products! SOP (time period, number specified?) are in place?	Part II-11.12, Annex 8-2.5

2 Lab Tour in Chemical and Physical-Chemical Laboratories

チェック項目	チェックNO	Requirement/要求事項	Questions／監査時の質問例	PIC/S GMP Guide NO.
Sampling（サンプリング）		以下の項目が定められていること ・サンプリングの一般方針 ・原材料のサンプリング場所 ・出発物質／包材サンプリング ・工程内（IPC）のサンプリング／中間体のサンプリング ・空気サンプリングシステム ・手順／記録 ・保管サンプル ・再サンプリング	サンプリングシステムの説明をしてください（認可，統計アプリケーション，サンプリング用具／区域） 採取したサンプルの数はどれくらいですか？ サンプリングはどのように行われますか？ 誰が行いますか？ サンプリングのためのSOPはありますか？ SOPには，容器，ラベル，機器の清掃などの詳細が含まれますか？ 分離したサンプリングエリアまたは保管エリアがありますか？ 交叉汚染／細菌汚染のリスクはどのように防止されていますか？ 工程管理／中間体サンプリングのシステム（SOP）は記載されていますか？ どのようなタイプのエアサンプラーが使用されていますか？その選定理由は何ですか？ サンプル量／テスト時間，使用培地，移動時間はどのくらいですか（SOP）？ 機器は校正されていますか？（プロトコールはありますか？） どのような殺菌処置が用いられていますか？ 機器を含めてどのようなサンプリング技術が採用されていますか？ 原材料と最終製品の残留サンプルの保管場所を見せてください。 SOP（サンプリングの間隔，数）がありますか？	

第III章 Audit Checklist for Plant/Laboratory Tour／プラント／ラボツアー実施のためのチェックリスト

チェック項目	チェックNO	Requirement/要求事項	Questions／監査時の質問例	PIC/S GMP Guide NO.
Handling of the samples（サンプルの取り扱い）	Ⅲ-38	The handling of the sample is defined.	How are the composite samples blended? How are (labelled, transferred, registered, distributed) samples for testing and contract testing handled (if applicable)? Is SOP(s) available? Do you have proper accountability of samples assessment? Are there used some contract facilities? Is responsibilities of CRO defined in Quality Agreement? Are the amount, time period and storage conditions defined at CRO? How long are sample stored prior testing? Show me the documentation.	Part Ⅱ-11.12, Annex 8-2, 3
		採取したサンプルの取扱いが定められていること	採取したサンプルはどのようにブレンドされていますか？ 契約試験機関で試験するサンプル（該当する場合）はどのように用意（ラベル，移送，登録，発送）されますか？ SOPは準備されていますか？ 検査されたサンプル評価の適切な説明責任をもっていますか？ 契約試験施設を利用していますか？ 契約試験施設の責任は契約に定義されていますか？ 契約試験施設でのサンプル必要量，期間，保管条件は定義されていますか？ 試験前にサンプルをどのくらいの時間，保管していますか？ 文書を見せてください	
Personnel for Sampling（サンプリング要員）	Ⅲ-39	training is being conducted.	Specifically training program for sampling is in-place?	Annex 8-1
		教育訓練が行われていること	サンプリング用の教育訓練プログラムはありますか？	

2 Lab Tour in Chemical and Physical-Chemical Laboratories

チェック項目	チェックNO	Requirement/要求事項	Questions/監査時の質問例	PIC/S GMP Guide NO.
Testing general（試験一般）	Ⅲ-40	QC system, Flow sheets, Methods, Contract testing, Re-testing are defined.	Are written documents available? Which types of testing are performed (e.g. microbiological, immunological, chemical etc.)? Specifying important steps? Which methods are used for testing? Standardized method (e.g. Pharmacopoeia), modified or developed in house? Which analyses are performed on contract facility (CRO)?	Part Ⅱ-11
		品質管理システム，フロー，試験法，委託試験，再試験が定められていること	文書はありますか？ どのタイプの試験（例えば，微生物学的，免疫学的，化学的等）が行われますか？ 重要なステップを指定しますか？ 試験に使用する試験法は標準化された方法（例えば薬局方）ですか？ それともインハウスのものですか？ どの分析試験が契約施設（CRO）で実施されていますか？	
Testing of Raw Materials（原材料試験）	Ⅲ-41	To have the written procedures.	Are Procedure(s) available? Do you have all Specification? Do the procedure comply with marketing authorization? Is Identity testing made for all container? Which materials are released on base of supplier's certificate? Are confirm with supplier's certificate approved/validated? Are acceptance limits specified?	Part Ⅱ-7.10, 7.20
		文書化された手順があること	手順はあり，利用可能ですか？ すべての規格はありますか？ この手順は承認要件に準拠していますか？ 確認試験はすべての容器に対して行われていますか？ どの原材料がサプライヤーの証明書（CoA）によって承認・合否判定されますか？ サプライヤーの証明書（CoA）が承認/検証されていますか？ 許容限界は規定されていますか？	

第III章 Audit Checklist for Plant/Laboratory Tour／プラント／ラボツアー実施のためのチェックリスト

チェック項目	チェックNO	Requirement/要求事項	Questions／監査時の質問例	PIC/S GMP Guide NO.
Testing of Intermediates（中間体の試験）	III-42	To have a system.	What is the testing strategy (extend, methods, parameters and limits used)? Which results are transferred into the final product protocol? Who takes samples for this testing?	Part II - 8.30, 8.31
		システムを有すること	試験戦略（範囲，方法，パラメータ，使用限界）は何ですか？ どの結果が最終製品プロトコールに記述されますか？ サンプルを採取するのは誰ですか？	
Testing of Final Products（最終製品の試験）	III-43	To have a sampling system handling samples correctly.	In which stages of processing are taken samples for final product testing? What kind of control is performed on final packages? What is the sampling plan (which norm is used)? How do you ensure the representatives of samples per batch? How do you handle the rests of final product samples (e.g. large volume containers)?	Part I - 6.11
		サンプリングのシステムがあり，サンプルを正しく取り扱っていること	どの段階で最終製品試験用のサンプルが採取されますか？ 最終パッケージではどのような管理が行われますか？ サンプリング計画の内容は何ですか（どの基準が使用されているか）？ バッチごとに代表サンプルであることをどのように確保しますか？ 最終製品サンプル（大容量容器など）の残りの部分はどのように扱いますか？	

チェック項目	チェック NO	Requirement/要求事項	Questions／監査時の質問例	PIC/S GMP Guide NO.
Stability Testing （保存安定性試験）	Ⅲ-44	Ongoing stability test, facility / equipment is appropriate.	Are Approach/policy define? Are Stability testing performed in place or contracted? Are full testing made? Are Critical parameters defined? What is the program (intervals, number of batches/products defined)? Are Analytical methods suitable? Which measures are taken in case if OOS results? Are appropriate storage stations available? Are storage sample dedicated, validated, labelled? Are thermometers and humidity meters calibrated? Is there continual monitoring of temperature and humidity? How are stored light sensitive materials? Is there an alarm system / is this documented?	Part Ⅱ - 11.5, Part Ⅰ - 6.26
		安定性試験，施設・機器が適切であること	取り組み／ポリシーは明記されていますか？ 保存安定性試験は，社内もしくは委託先で実施しましたか？ 完全なテストが行われていますか？ 重要なパラメータは定義されていますか？ プログラムの内容は何ですか（間隔，定義されたバッチ数/製品数）？ 分析方法は適切ですか？ OOSの結果が得られた場合，どの措置がとられますか？ 適切な保管場所がありますか？ 保管サンプルは専用で，検証され，ラベル付けされていますか？ 温度計と湿度計は校正されていますか？ 温度と湿度を継続的に監視していますか？ 光感受性の物質はどのように保管されていますか？ アラームシステムが備わっており，そのことが文書化されていますか？	

第III章 Audit Checklist for Plant/Laboratory Tour／プラント／ラボツアー実施のためのチェックリスト

チェック項目	チェックNO	Requirement/要求事項	Questions／監査時の質問例	PIC/S GMP Guide NO.
Validation of Test Methods（分析法バリデーション）	III-45	To have policy and procedures for validation according to ICH guidelines.	Is method validation a part of Validation Master Plan? Are General SOP on method validation available? Is Validation report formally approved by Quality Unit? Who approves? Is QA or QC? Do validation purposes specify in advance? Do Validation complete and document in each protocol for following parameters defined in ICH?: precision (System and method) intermediate precision - Accuracy - Specificity - Re-produceability - linearity (range) - limit of detection - limit of quantitation - robustness (including solution stability and filter compatibility) Are the following items documented in each SOP or protocol: - Acceptance criterion for each parameter defined and met - System suitability test procedure has been developed - Acceptance criterion for each system suitability parameter defined and met Where are raw data stored? Is there a SOP on method transfer?	Annex 15-9

チェック項目	チェックNO	Requirement/要求事項	Questions／監査時の質問例	PIC/S GMP Guide NO.
Validation of Test Methods （分析法バリデーション）		ICHガイドラインに則り，バリデーションポリシーがあり，手順を有すること	分析法バリデーションはバリデーションマスタープランの一部として準備されていますか？ 一般的なSOPは利用可能ですか？ バリデーション報告書は品質部門によって正式に承認されていますか？ 誰が承認するのですか？ QAまたはQCですか？ バリデーション目的はあらかじめ決めていますか？ ICHで定義されている以下のパラメータについて，バリデーションが完了し，各プロトコルで文書化していますか？ ・精度（システムと方法） ・中間精度 ・正確さ ・特異性 ・再現性 ・直線性（範囲） ・検出限界 ・定量限界 ・堅牢性（ソリューションの安定性とフィルターの互換性を含む） SOPまたはプロトコールごとに以下の事項が文書化されていますか？ ・各パラメータの合格基準が定義され，適合していること ・システム適合性試験手順が開発されていること ・各システム適合性合格基準が，決められ，適合していること 生データはどこに保存されますか？ 分析法移管のSOPはありますか？	

チェック項目	チェックNO	Requirement／要求事項	Questions／監査時の質問例	PIC/S GMP Guide NO.
Handling of test results （試験結果の取り扱い）	Ⅲ-46	To Confirm Transfer of raw data, Laboratory Management System (LIMS), Summary of raw data, Evaluation of test results, Trending analysis.	How are testing results (raw data) transferred into the summary protocol? Are analytical data reviewed by responsible person? How does responsible person review? Is the system validated? Was Training of operating personnel carried out? Is the access authorize and controlled? How? Is security of results ensured? What is your change control system? Who writes the final protocol? How and where are the raw data archived? Who is responsible for comments and evaluation of the results (QC manager)?	Part Ⅱ - 11.14
		生データの転記，試験室管理システム (LIMS)，生データのまとめ，試験結果の評価，トレンド分析を確認する	テスト結果（生データ）はどのように試験結果要約に転記されますか？ 分析データは責任者によって照査されていますか？ 責任者はどのように見直すのですか？ システムが検証されていますか？ 分析の訓練が行われましたか？ アクセスは許可され制御されていますか？どのようにですか？ 結果のセキュリティは保証されていますか？ 変更管理システムは整っていますか？ 最終的なプロトコールは誰が書いていますか？ 生データはどのようにアーカイブされていますか？ 結果のコメントと評価を担当するのは誰ですか（QCマネージャー）？	
Failures – Out of Specification (OOS) test results （規格外試験結果の取り扱い）	Ⅲ-47	To confirm the following items; • System/OOS • Laboratory errors operator, equipment) Process/Procedure related errors • Evaluation of OOS results • Test results invalidation・reject • Corrective action	Is there a SOP for OOS result investigation? How is your reporting procedure? QA is involved? What is the procedure on decision related to OOS? Are reasons of OOS defined? How are test results invalidated? Who can invalidate the testing results? How do a corrective action implement?	Part Ⅱ - 11.15

チェック項目	チェック NO	Requirement／要求事項	Questions／監査時の質問例	PIC/S GMP Guide NO.
Failures – Out of Specification (OOS) test results （規格外試験結果の取り扱い）		以下の事項を確認すること ・OOSの取り扱い手順 ・ラボエラー ・試験者，機器のエラー ・試験法に依存するエラー ・OOS結果評価 ・試験結果の破棄 ・是正	OOS結果調査のためのSOPはありますか？ 報告手順はどのようになっていますか？ QAは関係していますか？ OOSに関連する決定にはどのような手続きがありますか？ OOSの理由は定義されていますか？ 試験結果はどのように無効になるのですか？ 試験結果を無効にすることができるのは誰ですか？ 是正措置はどのように実施されていますか？	
Failures- Retesting and Resampling （再試験・再サンプリング）	Ⅲ-48	Procedure and re-testing program and criteria for re-sampling is defined.	How often can a retest be performed? How many times could be testing repeated (testing into compliance)? What are criteria for re-sampling (e.g. if the sample was not representative)? Who can allow re-sampling?	Part Ⅱ- 11.15
		手順および再試験と再サンプリングの許可要件が定められていること	再試験はどのくらいの頻度で行うことができますか？ 何回，再試験でますか（コンプライアンスのテスト） 再サンプリングの基準は何ですか（例：サンプルが代表でない場合）？ 再サンプリングを許可できるのは誰ですか？	
Release of test results／analytical reports／certification （出荷判定試験，分析報告書，CoA）	Ⅲ-49	The procedure of issuing the test results and preparation of the report are defined.	Do you have appropriate SOPs? Who's responsible for review, decisions, conclusions and formal release of batch? How much is the validity of analytical results taken into the consideration? Who prepares and approves Summary Report (QC manager)? Who approves Certificate of analyses? QA involved?	Part Ⅱ- 11.43
		試験結果の発行の手順や報告書の作成が定められていること	SOPは備わっていますか？ 誰がバッチのレビュー，判定および正式出荷承認を担当していますか？ 分析結果の妥当性はどの程度考慮されますか？ 要約レポートを作成し承認するのは誰ですか？ QCマネージャーですか？ 誰がCoAを承認しますか？ 関連するQAですか？	

Microbiological Laboratories／微生物試験室

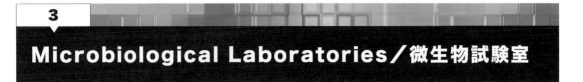

微生物試験室

微生物試験特有の項目が存在するので，それらに着眼することを忘れないように監査を行うこと。

チェック項目	チェックNO	Requirement／要求事項	Questions／監査時の質問例	PIC/S GMP Guide NO.
Premises（施設）	Ⅲ-50	To confirm the following items; • Areas / Sterility testing area • Areas for positive control tests and fertility testing • Air supply and ventilation system in microbiological laboratory • Area of preparation • Washing room	How do you design laboratory area to meet guideline/requirement? Where do you carry out are sterility tests? In isolator or other? How do you assess the efficiency against microbiological contamination during aseptic operations? Do you have appropriate instructions for access into the critical areas? Is there area for positive tests/fertility testing separate from areas where product is tested? Is the system for microbiological laboratories properly designed? Show me the schematic drawing. Is the ventilation system/line separated from other areas? What are the pressure differentials (e.g. airlock-test room)? Are there visual alarms? Where do you prepare materials for aseptic operations? Where do you prepare culture media for testing? Is there any segregated area/room for manipulation with culture media? How and where are decontaminated materials from microbiological testing? Is there some segregation of washing area to the clean and non clean part?	Part Ⅱ - 4.16, 4.60

3 Microbiological Laboratories

チェック項目	チェックNO	Requirement/要求事項	Questions／監査時の質問例	PIC/S GMP Guide NO.
Premises（施設）		以下を確認すること ・通常区域／無菌テスト区域 ・陽性確認試験と増殖テストのエリア ・微生物試験室における空気供給と換気システム ・準備室 ・洗浄室	試験室は，要求項に適合するように，どのように設計しましたか？ 無菌テストはどこで実施していますか？ アイソレータですか他の施設ですか？ 無菌操作中の微生物汚染防止の効率をどのように評価していますか？ 重要管理区域へのアクセスに適切な指示がありますか？ 製品がテストされている地域と離れた場所・施設で陽性試験／増殖試験を行いますか？ 微生物試験室のシステムは適切に設計されていますか？ 配管図面を見せてください 換気システム／ラインは他の試験区域から分離されていますか？ 差圧（エアロック試験室など）は，いくつに設定されていますか？ アラームは備えていますか？ 無菌操作のために資材はどこで準備しますか？ 試験のための培養培地はどこで用意していますか？ 培養培地を操作するための隔離区画/部屋はありますか？ どのように，どこで，微生物試験で汚染された部材等を除菌しますか？ 汚染されたものと汚染されていないものを分離して洗浄する施設はありますか？	

チェック項目	チェックNO	Requirement/要求事項	Questions／監査時の質問例	PIC/S GMP Guide NO.
Equipment（機器）	III-51	To confirm the following items; • Isolators used for the sterility testing • Incubators • Autoclave • Sterilization by autoclave • HEPA Filters (validation/maintenance)	Do you complete IQ, OQ, PQ? Show me the results (report). Show me the results of leak test in general (same as Lamina Air Flow). Show me the document involving the temperature mapping. Do you conduct Calibration of instrument for measurements of humidity? Show us the results of validation of Autoclave(cold points, replacing cycles number, stacking). How do you maintain/re-qualify autoclave? What is the quality of steam (quality SPECIFICATION)? What kinds of control test are performed in the steam? What equipment is sterilized? How is equipment sterilized? Are there raw data available (cycle/temperature records)? How are goods handled, which have been run a failed cycle (SOP)? What ways do you have to ensure the integrity of filters (HEPA)? How long is the frequency of their replacement? How do you ensure there is no leakage after replacement?	Annex 1-43〜55

3 Microbiological Laboratories

チェック項目	チェックNO	Requirement/要求事項	Questions／監査時の質問例	PIC/S GMP Guide NO.
Equipment（機器）		以下の項目を確認すること ・滅菌試験のため使用するアイソレーター ・培養器 ・オートクレーブ ・オートクレーブを用いての滅菌 ・HEPAフィルターのバリデーション・維持	IQ, OQ, PQを完了していますか？ 結果を見せてください（IQ,OQ,PQの報告書，QA承認済み）。 リークテストの結果を見せてください（もしくはラミナーエアフローの確認試験）。 温度マッピングを行った結果を見せてください。 湿度測定機器の校正を行っていますか？ オートクレーブのバリデーション結果を見せてください（コールドポイント，入れ替え回数，積重ね段数を表示してください）。 オートクレーブをどのように維持／再評価しますか？ スチームの規格品質はどのようになっていますか？ 蒸気についてどのような品質管理試験が行われますか？ どのような機器が滅菌対象ですか？ 機器はどのように滅菌されていますか？ 生データ（サイクル／温度記録）がありますか？ 不良なサイクルで殺菌が行われたとき，被殺菌物はどのように処理されますか？ フィルター（HEPA）の完全性試験をどのように行いますか？ フィルター（HEPA）の交換頻度はどのくらいですか？ 交換後の漏れをどのように確認していますか？	
	Ⅲ-52	To confirm the following items; • Colony counter unit • Particle counter • Microscope	Do you do calibration? How do you do calibration? Show me the document on qualification. Which type colony counter do you use? Was that instrument qualified?	Annex 1-57
		以下を確認すること ・コロニー測定器 ・微粒子測定器 ・顕微鏡	校正を行っていますか？ どのように校正しますか？ 適格性試験報告書を見せてください。 どのタイプのコロニーカウンターを使用していますか？ その機器は適格性確認されていましたか？	

3 微生物試験室

チェック項目	チェックNO	Requirement/ 要求事項	Questions／監査時の質問例	PIC/S GMP Guide NO.
Testing materials （試験材料）	Ⅲ-53	To confirm the following items; • Settle plates • Culture media (kind, purpose) • Culture collection/ Reference. standards	What media type do you adapt for incubation? Have the plates been irradiated? How long are plates exposure and how is it calculated (dryness!)? Is there tested each batch (growth promotion, selectivity, sterility)? Is there an agreement available on shipment (plates) of prepared media? How is shipping validation performed? How do you guarantee that shipment conditions are kept constant? How do you store the reagents and standard strains used for the identification? Show me the inventory. Are identifications of strains carried out on arrival? Expiration was indicated on labels?	Part Ⅱ- 11.23
		以下の事項を確認すること ・静置培地 ・培地（種類・適用範囲） ・微生物株保存機関，標準株	細菌および酵母の培養に適した培地は，どの種類ですか？ プレートは，放射線照射されていますか？ プレートの（大気）曝露時間はどのくらいですか，それはどのように計測されますか？ 各バッチは増殖促進，選択性，無菌性が試験されていますか？ 準備された培地の出荷（プレート）で利用できる契約はありますか？ 出荷バリデーションはどのように行われますか？ 出荷条件が一定に保たれていることをどのように保証しますか？ 同定に使用した試薬や標準株はどのように保管していますか？ 在庫を見せてください。 到着時に菌株の同定が行われていますか？ 有効期限はラベルに記載されていますか？	

3 Microbiological Laboratories

チェック項目	チェックNO	Requirement/要求事項	Questions／監査時の質問例	PIC/S GMP Guide NO.
Protective garments （更衣）	Ⅲ-54	Preparation on gowning and Use in performance.	How do you wash gowns and/or sterilize? Which protective garments are used by operators at sterility testing? Are protective garments suitable for intended use? Are the laboratory coats located in appropriate manner? Do you have Instructions for use? Do you train operators in advance? What standard for micro assays is used?	Part Ⅱ-3.21
		保護服が準備され有用であること	保護服の洗浄・滅菌をどのように行いますか？ 滅菌試験の際にどの保護服を作業者は使用しますか？ 保護服は意図された用途に適していますか？ ラボ用保護服は適切な方法で配置されていますか？ 使用説明書はありますか？ 事前に作業者を訓練していますか？ 微生物試験にはどの標準保護服が使用されていますか？	

第III章 Audit Checklist for Plant/Laboratory Tour／プラント／ラボツアー実施のためのチェックリスト

チェック項目	チェックNO	Requirement/要求事項	Questions／監査時の質問例	PIC/S GMP Guide NO.
Microbiological Testing (product) (製品の微生物試験)	III-55	To confirm the following items; • Incubation • Positive controls • Negative controls • Bioburden • Micro-organism – identification	Show us the limits of incubation. What is the incubation time and temperature? What is the frequency of observation of sample during incubation? Do you have records (registration/incubation)? Which micro-organisms are used? Do you have the procedure for Precultures? Which controls do you have? How often do you perform positive controls and why? Do you perform negative product controls? Show me The SOP (number of containers/samples). Do you define limits and use in production/in process controls? Does bioburden IPC'S show the worst case conditions? Which system do you use to identify?	Part II - 11.23
		以下の項目を確認すること ・培養 ・ポジティブコントロール ・ネガティブコントロール ・バイオバーデン ・微生物の同定	培養の限界を教えてください 培養時間と温度は？ 培養中のサンプルの観察頻度はどのくらいですか？ 記録（登録／培養）がありますか？ どの微生物が使用されていますか？ 予備培養の手順はありますか？ どのような管理を行っていましたか？ どのくらいの頻度でポジティブコントロールを用いますか？なぜですか？ ネガティブコントロールを行っていますか？ 容器数／サンプル数を記述したSOPを見せてください 生産／プロセス管理で，限界，使用目的を決めていますか？ バイオバーデンIPCはワーストケースに対して行われましたか？ どのシステムを使って同定していますか？	

3　Microbiological Laboratories

チェック項目	チェック NO	Requirement/要求事項	Questions／監査時の質問例	PIC/S GMP Guide NO.
Microbiological testing (Environmental) (微生物試験, 環境試験)	Ⅲ-56	To confirm the following items; • Sampling location • Swabs • Settlement plate • Contact plates • Limits for microbiological testing	How is monitoring performed at rest/in operation? How is the frequency? How do you test verification performed? Is the monitoring involved in validation plan? Are there available documents on pre-qualification/re-qualification? How do you select location / sampling sites? How do you determine the worst case? Water system/area are included to determine the worst case? How do you handle deviations? Do you do Validation? Which/what swabbing techniques do you use? Which media used? What is the method, time exposure, surface area/limits and recovery rate?	Annex 15 -10.7～12
		以下の項目を確認すること ・サンプリング場所 ・スワブ試験 ・沈下板 ・接触試験 ・微生物限度試験	モニタリングは，休止中／運転中にどのように行われますか？ 頻度はどれくらいですか？ 適格性はどのように検証されますか？ モニタリングは検証計画に含まれていますか？ 事前適格性／再適格性に関する文書がありますか？ どのように場所／サンプリングサイトが選択されていますか？ どのようにワーストケースを決定しますか？ ワーストケースを判断するのに水システム／範囲が考慮されていますか？ 逸脱をどのように扱いますか？バリデーションをしますか？ どのスワブ法を採用しますか？ どの培地を使用しましたか？ 方法，曝露時間，表面積／限度および回収率はどのくらいですか？	

第 IV 章

Audit Checklist on Prevention for Cross Contamination／交叉汚染対策のためのチェックリスト

　本章で示すチェックリストは，I～III章とは異なり，特定の施設／品質システム等の固有のものに対する監査に焦点を当ててはいない。ここでは，GMPの3原則の1つである「汚染および品質低下を防止すること」を取り上げ，リスク分析・対策の取り組みを監査する手法を解説することを趣旨としている。

　従来，監査員は，個々の機器，手順に対して質問，文書記録の照査を行っていた。かつては品質に影響を及ぼす重大な要因は品質の不安定さであったが，機器・品質管理が近代化とともに飛躍的に改善され，近年のRisk based GMPにおいては交叉汚染・混同が最大の品質影響要素と考えられる。FDA，EMAの査察においても，査察官は交叉汚染防止と混同防止に多く注目して，査察を行うといわれている。

　I～III章では全体の監査の流れを説明する意味合いが強かったため，チェックリストの表の中に「チェック項目」を示していたが，本章ではその欄は割愛し，「1.全体，2.設備・機器，3.一般組織管理，4.キャンペーン製造，5.機器の洗浄，6.洗浄バリデーション・ベリフィケーション，7.従業員・教育訓練」の7つのチェックリストとした。

1 Overview on Cross Contamination／全体

リスクベースアプローチ

全体的な事項として，リスクベースアプローチが基本となる。汚染リスクの大きさをしっかりと把握し，それに見合った対策が各所で取られているかといったことの確認が基本となる。

チェックNO	PIC/S Requirement／PIC/Sの要求項目	Questions／監査時の質問例	PIC/S GMP Guide NO.
IV-1	Quality risk management is a systematic process for the assessment, control, communication and review of risks to the quality of the drug (medicinal) product across the product lifecycle.	Do you define and document your Risk management system and related measurements; e.g., risk assessment, periodical review of risk management system	Annex 20-15
	品質リスク管理は，医薬品のライフサイクルにわたる医薬品の品質へのリスク評価，管理，コミュニケーション，レビューのためのシステム的な工程である	リスク管理と関連する手順・基準を定め，文書化していますか？　例えばリスク評価，リスク管理システムの定期的レビュー	
IV-2	Quality Management is a wide-ranging concept, which covers all matters, which individually or collectively influence the quality of a product.	Do you complete risk assessment and take an action for mitigation of risk contamination, cross contamination and/or mixed up of drug (medicinal) product across the product lifecycle?	Part I -1.1, 3-principle
	品質マネジメントは，個別的または集合的に製品の品質に影響するすべての事項をカバーする広範なコンセプトである	医薬品のライフサイクルにわたる品質へのリスク（汚染，交叉汚染，混同）を評価して，軽減策を講じていますか？	
IV-3	The measures to prevent cross-contamination should be commensurate with the risks. Quality Risk Management principles should be used to assess and control the risks.	Do you allocate time on inspection to evaluate the risks the level of sharing of premises/ equipment / utilities etc. that takes place?	Part I -3.6
	製造施設の適切な設計と運用により，すべての製品の交叉汚染を防止すること。交叉汚染を防止するための措置は，リスクに見合ったものでなければならない	施設／設備／ユーティリティなどの共有化のリスクを評価するために調査する時間を割り当てていますか？	
IV-4	Depending of the level of risk, it may be necessary to dedicate premises and equipment for manufacturing and/or packaging operations to control the risk presented by some medicinal products.	Do you evaluate any hazards presented by neighboring facilities or other buildings in the facility relevant to your facility and building (e.g. Air Handling Units (AHU) outlets and intake locations)?	Part I -3.6
	リスクのレベルに応じて，いくつかの医薬品に起因するリスクを管理するために，製造および／または包装作業のために施設および設備を専用化することが必要な場合がある	施設内の近隣施設または他の建物（例えば，エアハンドリングユニット（AHU）吸入および排出場所）による危険性が検査されていますか？	

1 Overview on Cross Contamination

チェック NO	PIC/S Requirement／PIC/Sの要求項目	Questions／監査時の質問例	PIC/S GMP Guide NO.
IV-5	Documentation may exist in a variety of forms, including paper-based, electronic or photographic media. The main objective of the system of documentation utilized must be to establish, control, monitor and record all activities which directly or indirectly impact on all aspects of the quality of medicinal products.	Do you (your site) have an adequately documented policy and strategy for implementation for control of cross-contamination that reflects the hazards associated with products made or planned to be made? Does the policy and strategy clearly state any product classes manufactured or excluded from manufacture at your site or clarify circumstances under which higher hazard products may be introduced?	Part Ⅰ-4 principle, 5.18.
	文書は，種々の形態（紙ベース，電子媒体，写真媒体を含む）で存在する。文書化システムを活用する主な目的は，医薬品の品質のすべての面に直接または間接的に影響を与えるすべての活動を確立し，管理し，モニターし，記録することである	作成または計画された，製品に関連する危険性を反映する交叉汚染管理のための適切な文書化された方針と戦略がありますか？ 方針および戦略は，製造された製品または現場での製造から除外された製品の分類を明確に定めていますか？ またはより高い危険性の製品が導入される可能性のある状況下での環境の浄化を定めていますか？	
IV-6	Where a worst case product approach is used as a cleaning validation model, a scientific rationale should be provided for the selection of the worst case product and the impact of new products to the site assessed. Criteria for determining the worst case may include solubility, cleanability, toxicity, and potency.	Do you have the procedure to control for New Product Introduction with respect to cross-contamination control?	Annex 15-10
	ワーストケースの製品を用いて洗浄バリデーションモデルとする場合，ワーストケースの製品の選択と製造サイトへの評価の新製品の影響について科学的根拠が提供されるべきである。ワーストケースを決定するための基準には，溶解度，洗浄の容易性，毒性，および効力が含まれ得る	交叉汚染管理に関して，新製品導入を管理する手順はありますか？	
IV-7	Layout and design must aim to minimize the risk of errors and permit effective cleaning and maintenance in order to avoid cross-contamination, build-up of dust or dirt and, in general, any adverse effect on the quality of products.	Do you have the procedure to control for retiring or re-designation of equipment / facilities with cross-contamination control in mind?	Part Ⅰ-3 principle
	配置および設計は，交叉汚染，ほこりや汚れの蓄積，製品の品質への悪影響を避けるために，エラーのリスクを最小限に抑え，効果的な洗浄とメンテナンスを行うことを目指す必要がある	交叉汚染防止を考慮した機器／施設の廃止または再設計のための適切な管理手順はありますか？	
IV-8	Contamination of a starting material or of a product by another material or product should be prevented.	Do you identify all products including all products currently manufactured and/or stored at site (for any country/market), legacy products which have been manufactured in recent years and non-medicinal products as well as raw material?	Part Ⅰ-5.18
	他の原材料または製品による，出発原料または製品の汚染を回避しなければならない	製造場所で製造・保管されているすべての製品（すべての国／市場），近年製造された長期収載品，非医薬品，原材料を含むすべての製品が特定されていますか？	

第IV章 Audit Checklist on Prevention for Cross Contamination／交叉汚染対策のためのチェックリスト

チェックNO	PIC/S Requirement／PIC/Sの要求項目	Questions／監査時の質問例	PIC/S GMP Guide NO.
IV-9	Depending of the level of risk, it may be necessary to dedicate premises and equipment for manufacturing and/or packaging operations to control the risk presented by some medicinal products.	Do you consider that the products manufactured in shared facilities will be a significant hazard that may present a cross-contamination concern?	Part I - 3.6
	リスクのレベルに応じて，いくつかの医薬品に起因するリスクを管理するために，製造および/または包装作業のために施設および設備を専用化することが必要な場合がある	共有施設で製造された製品は，交叉汚染の懸念を呈する重大なハザードになると考えていますか？	
IV-10	The significance of this risk varies with the nature of the contaminant and that of the product being contaminated.	Do you identify the hazards associated with the products adequately?	Part I - 5.18, Annex 15-10.6
	リスクの重要性は，汚染物質の性質と汚染された製品の性質によって異なる	医薬品に関連するハザードは十分に識別されていますか？	
IV-11	Contamination of a starting material or of a product by another material or product should be prevented. This risk of accidental cross-contamination resulting from the uncontrolled release of dust, gases, vapors, aerosols, genetic material or organisms from active substances, other materials (starting or in-process), and products in process, from residues on equipment, and from operators' clothing should be assessed.	Do you consider that the extent and reliability of the manufacturer's product knowledge are commensurate with the hazard? For contract manufacturers – is there sufficient knowledge on site about the products they manufacture to ensure cross-contamination can be controlled adequately?	Part I - 5.18, Annex 13-5, Annex 15-10.6
	出発材料または製品が他の材料または製品によって汚染されるのを防ぐ必要がある。ダスト，ガス，蒸気，エアゾル，遺伝物質または（微）生物が活性物質，その他の物質（開始または処理中），および処理中の製品，装置の残留物からの制御されない放出に起因する，また作業員の衣服から偶発的な交叉汚染のリスクを評価する必要がある	製造元の医薬品知識の範囲と信頼性は，ハザードと釣り合っていると考えていますか？ 契約製造業者（CMO）は，交叉汚染を適切に管理して，医薬品を製造するための十分な知識がありますか？	
IV-12	Limits for the carryover of product residues should be based on a toxicological evaluation.	Do you identify the hazards in an appropriate manner (e.g. via Permitted Daily Exposure (PDE) approach or other appropriate compliance/safety references)?	Annex 15-10.6, Part I - 5.18
	前製造由来の残留基準は，毒性学的評価に基づくものでなければならない	ハザードは適切な手方で特定しましたか？（例：1日最大摂取許容量（PDE），その他の適切なコンプライアンス／安全基準）	

チェック NO	PIC/S Requirement／PIC/Sの要求項目	Questions／監査時の質問例	PIC/S GMP Guide NO.
IV-13	People in responsible positions should have specific duties recorded in written job descriptions and adequate authority to carry out their responsibilities. Their duties may be delegated to designated deputies of a satisfactory qualification level.	Do you have a scientific basis for the hazard assessment? Does the person performing the hazard assessment have appropriate education, training and experience? Is there appropriate resource available to carry out the hazard assessment? If hazard assessment is an outsourced activity, is it adequately controlled?	Part I - 2.3, 2.10, 2.11, 5.18
	責任ある職位にある者は，職務記述書に記録された特定の職責を有し，職責を実施する適切な権限を有すること。職責は，十分な資格レベルの指定された代理人に委任することができる	ハザード評価の科学的根拠はありますか？ ハザード評価を実施している人は適切な教育訓練を受け，経験を持っていますか？ ハザード評価を実施するのに適切なリソースがありますか？ （ハザード評価を外注している場合）適切に管理されていますか？	
IV-14	Documents should be designed, prepared, reviewed, and distributed with care	Do you have a procedure on hazard assessment and is it approved?	Part I - 4.1, 4.2
	文書は注意して設計し，作成し，照査し，配布すること	ハザード評価の手順を有しており，承認されていますか？	
IV-15	Documents containing instructions should be approved, signed and dated by appropriate and authorized persons.	Do you adequately document the hazard assessment been and conduct in accordance with the procedure?	Part I - 4.3, 4.8
	指図を含む文書は，権限を持つ者が承認し，署名し，日付を入れること	ハザードの評価は，手順に従って適切に実施・文書化されていますか？	
IV-16	The level of effort, formality and documentation of the Quality Risk Management process is commensurate with the level of risk.	Is your level of the assessment, control, communication and review the detail/adequate to present the level of hazard and any conclusions in the assessment document? Note: Auditors may need to refer to toxicology experts within their own agency.	Part I - 1.12, 1.13, 3.6
	品質リスクマネジメントのプロセスについての労力レベル，社内手続きの正式度および文書化の程度は，リスクの程度に相応する	評価報告書中の結論，ハザードのレベルを表すのに貴社の評価・管理・コミュニケーション・照査のレベルは，適切かつ詳細なレベルですか？ 注：監査者は，規定当局内の毒物学の専門家を参照する必要があるかもしれない	

チェック NO	PIC/S Requirement／PIC/S の要求項目	Questions／監査時の質問例	PIC/S GMP Guide NO.
IV-17	Quality Risk Management is a systematic process for the assessment, control, communication and review of risks to the quality of the medicinal product. It can be applied both proactively and retrospectively.	Do you have an adequate QRM approach for identification and management of contamination risk? Do you document a procedure and output, adequately? Does the QRM process include: • Assessment (Identification, analysis & evaluation), • Control, • Communication, and • Review Is the manufacturer's approach robust, scientifically valid and adequately addresses the hazard presented by the product?	Part I - 1.12, 1.13, 3.6
	品質リスクマネジメントは，医薬品の品質へのリスクの評価，管理，伝達および照査のための体系的なプロセスである。事前対応としても回顧的にも適用することができる	汚染リスクの特定と管理には，適切なQRMアプローチがありますか？ 手続きがあり，適切に文書化されて出力されていますか？ QRMプロセスには以下が含まれますか？ ・評価（識別，分析および評価） ・管理 ・コミュニケーション ・照査 製造業者のアプローチは頑健で，科学的に有効であり，製品が持つハザードに適切に対応していますか？	
IV-18	Cross-contamination should be prevented by attention to design of the premises and equipment.	If your facility has segregated grouped products, then how do you control the cross- contamination risk? Within the group (e.g. hormonal products, or different cytotoxics in the same facility) is there a scientific rationale for the grouping of the products and for the controls exercised in such areas? Is risk control adequate to address the potential impact outside the group/area?	Part I - 5.19
	交叉汚染は，施設や設備の設計に注意を払うことによって防止する必要がある	施設がグループ化された製品を分離している場合，交叉汚染のリスクはどのように管理していますか？ グループ内（例えば，ホルモン様医薬品，または同じ施設内の異種の細胞毒性物質）には，製品のグループ分けおよびそのような領域で訓練された管理に関する科学的根拠がありますか？ グループ／エリア外への潜在的な影響に対処するために，リスクコントロールは適切ですか？	

チェック NO	PIC/S Requirement／PIC/Sの要求項目	Questions／監査時の質問例	PIC/S GMP Guide NO.
IV-19	The evaluation of the risk to quality is based on scientific knowledge, experience with the process and ultimately links to the protection of the patient.	Do you investigate the risk management study adequately to address potential failure in controls? Do you have an adequate strategy to address failures including • Anticipating human failures to follow systems (especially work which is manually performed) • Equipment breakdown • Failure of primary containment • Power outages affecting AHU • Product/material spills • Accidental exposure • Rework/reprocessing occurring out of sync with the campaign manufacturing plan?	Part Ⅰ-1.12, 1.13, 3.6
	品質へのリスクの評価は，科学的知見，工程の経験に基づくものであり，最終的に患者保護に帰結する	リスク管理研究では，管理に潜む失敗に対して適切に対処していますか？ 失敗に対処するための適切な戦略を持っていますか？ ・ヒューマンエラーを予測すること（特に手作業で行われる作業） ・機器の故障 ・一次封じ込めの失敗 ・AHUの作動に影響を及ぼす停電 ・製品／材料のこぼれ ・偶発的な曝露 ・キャンペーン製造計画と同期がとれない再加工／再処理の発生	
IV-20	Besides the basic training on the theory and practice of the Pharmaceutical Quality System and Good Manufacturing Practice, newly recruited personnel should receive training appropriate to the duties assigned to them. Continuing training should also be given, and its practical effectiveness should be periodically assessed.	Can you show us any evidence / demonstrate that it has the skills, knowledge, competency, controls (including equipment, facility design, people skills, organization, etc.) to manufacture the products in question in a shared facility?	Part Ⅰ-2.10, 2.11
	医薬品品質システムならびにGMPの理論および実践に関する基本的な教育訓練以外に，新規に採用された人員は，割り当てられた職責に応じた適切な教育訓練を受けること。継続的な教育訓練も実施し，その実効性を定期的に評価すること	共用施設において生産することに問題のある製品を製造するスキル，知識，能力，管理（設備，設備設計，人材スキル，組織などを含む）を有することの証拠を有していますか？	
IV-21	Quality Risk Management is a systematic process for the assessment, control, communication and review of risks to the quality of the medicinal product.	Do you communicate the risks adequately to all relevant personnel?	Part Ⅰ-1.12, 1.13
	品質リスクマネジメントは，医薬品の品質へのリスクの評価，管理，伝達および照査のための体系的なプロセスである	リスクは関係者全員に適切に伝えられていますか（共有化されていますか）？	

第IV章 Audit Checklist on Prevention for Cross Contamination／交叉汚染対策のためのチェックリスト

チェック NO	PIC/S Requirement／PIC/Sの要求項目	Questions／監査時の質問例	PIC/S GMP Guide NO.
IV-22	Measures to prevent cross-contamination and their effectiveness should be reviewed periodically according to set procedures. Following implementation, and where appropriate, an evaluation of the effectiveness of change should be carried out to confirm that the change has been successful.	Do you define the frequency of periodic review? If new data are available or the original hazard analysis is wonder to be appropriate, is your defined frequency adequate to determine? Is there a mechanism to ensure follow through from pharmacovigilance data analysis? Do you take new scientific knowledge into account?	Part I - 5.22, Annex 15-11.7
	交叉汚染を防止する手段およびその有効性を，所定の手順書に従って定期的にレビューすること。実施後，適切な場合には，変更が有効であることを確認するために，変更の有効性評価が行われなければならない	定期照査の頻度は決めていますか？ 元のハザード分析が現在も適切かどうかが疑問になった，もしくは新しく入手可能なデータを入手した場合，定めた定期照査の頻度・間隔は適切ですか？ 薬物モニタリングのデータ分析から確実に結論を導く機能はありますか？ 新しい科学知識を取り込んでいますか？	
IV-23	Following implementation, and where appropriate, an evaluation of the effectiveness of change should be carried out to confirm that the change has been successful.	Do you take any changes to the product portfolio into account when reviewing the use of the hazard analysis? Examples include introduction of products associated with a potentially more vulnerable patient group or change in route of administration such as liquids for external use to liquids for internal use, introduction of intravenous products, and change to particle size (e.g. micronized form), new target species.	Annex 15-11.1, 11.7
	変更実施後，適切な場合には，変更が有効であることを確認するために，変更の有効性の評価が行われなければならない	ハザード分析の使用を検討する際に，製品ポートフォリオの変更が考慮されていますか？ 例としては，潜在的により脆弱な患者群に関連する製品の導入，または液外用剤液の内服剤への投与系の変更，静脈注の導入，および粒子サイズ（例えば微粉化）の変更，新しい標的種	
IV-24	Quality Management is a wide-ranging concept, which covers all matters, which individually or collectively influence the quality of a product. It is the sum total of the organized arrangements made with the objective of ensuring that medicinal products are of the quality required for their intended use.	Do you consider your control systems would be robust enough to ensure detection and identification of cross-contamination issues (e.g. where appropriate do the manufacturer's procedures consider that cross-contamination could be the possible cause for complaints and out of specification results)?	Part I - 1.1
	品質マネジメントは，個別的または集合的に製品の品質に影響するすべての事項をカバーする広範なコンセプトである。医薬品がその使用目的に求められる品質を具備することを保証する目的で作られた，組織化された取決めの集大成である	交叉汚染の問題検出と同定を確実に行うための管理システムは十分に堅牢であると考えていますか（例えば，交叉汚染が苦情の原因とOOSの結果になる可能性があることを適切に検討する手順がありますか）？	

チェック NO	PIC/S Requirement／PIC/Sの要求項目	Questions／監査時の質問例	PIC/S GMP Guide NO.
IV-25	The output/results of the risk management process should be reviewed to take into account new knowledge and experience. Once a quality risk management process has been initiated, that process should continue to be utilized for events that might impact the original quality risk management decision, whether these events are planned or unplanned.	Do you periodically review of the controls established in the risk assessment to ensure ongoing suitability? Do you take any changes to manufacturing process/ infrastructure/ equipment/ utilities/ etc. take into account the potential impact on cross-contamination?	Annex 20-31, 32, Part Ⅰ- 1.12, 1.13, Annex 15-11.4
	リスク管理プロセスの成果／結果は，新しい知識と経験を考慮して見直されるべきである。品質リスクマネジメントプロセスが開始されると，そのプロセスが計画されているか計画されていないかにかかわらず，元の品質リスクマネジメントの決定に影響を与える可能性がある事象に対して，そのプロセスを引き続き活用すること	継続的な適合性を確保するために，リスクアセスメントで確立された管理手法の定期的な照査・見直しを行っていますか？ 製造プロセス／施設／設備／ユーティリティ／その他への変更は，交叉汚染の潜在的影響を考慮していますか？	

2 Premises, Equipment／設備・機器

設計思想が反映されているか

　交叉汚染防止は，設備・機器などハード面での対応が必要な部分も大きい。洗浄性などを考慮して設計されているかといったことの確認とともに，運用する製造所の意識が伴っていることも監査の中でチェックする。

チェックNO	PIC/S Requirement／PIC/Sの要求項目	Questions／監査時の質問例	PIC/S GMP Guide NO.
IV-26	Cross-contamination should be prevented for all products by appropriate design and operation of manufacturing facilities. The measures to prevent cross-contamination should be commensurate with the risks. Quality Risk Management principles should be used to assess and control the risks.	Do you have appropriate design measures, in terms of premises, for prevention of cross-contamination and are they consistent with the output of the QRM process? Do you consider the qualification of the facility support the cross-contamination strategy and design philosophy?	Part I - 1.12, 1.13, 3.1, 3.6, 3.7, 5.19
	製造施設の適切な設計と運用により，すべての製品の交叉汚染を防止すること。交叉汚染を防止するための措置は，リスクに見合ったものでなければならない	交叉汚染の防止のための適切な設計措置を講じていますか？それがQRMプロセスの成果と一致していますか？ 施設の適格性が交叉汚染防止戦略と設計思想をサポートしていますか？	
IV-27	Premises should preferably be laid out in such a way as to allow the production to take place in areas connected in a logical order corresponding to the sequence of the operations and to the requisite cleanliness levels. In cases where dust is generated, specific provisions should be taken to avoid cross-contamination and facilitate cleaning.	Do you design the premises including siting of equipment facilitate to be good containment relative to the type of products/materials handled? Particularly where there may be open handling of materials.	Part I - 3.6～3.8, 3.14
	作業の流れおよび必要な清浄度レベルに応じた論理的な順序で連結した区域において製造が行われるよう，建物を設計することが望ましい。 埃が発生する場合は，交叉汚染を回避して清掃を行いやすくする特別な予防措置を講じること	設備の配置を含め，施設は取り扱う製品／材料のタイプに関連付けて良好な封じ込めを容易にする設計ですか？ 特に，原材料を開封する場所・区域	
IV-28	Cross-contamination should be prevented by attention to design of the premises and equipment.	Do you have adequate structural design provisions such as air locks, air showers and segregated or enhanced gowning/de-gowning areas been incorporated and meet desired effectiveness? Where appropriate, do you have dedicated utilities such as AHU, water systems, compressed air/gas and effluent/waste streams, for different products been incorporated? Could back flow in utilities cause a risk of cross-contamination?	Part I - 5.19

2 Premises, Equipment

チェックNO	PIC/S Requirement／PIC/Sの要求項目	Questions／監査時の質問例	PIC/S GMP Guide NO.
IV-29	交叉汚染は，機器設備の設計に注意を払うことによって防止すること	エアロック，エアシャワー，分離されたまたは高性能化した更衣区域など適切な構造設計規定が組み込まれ，期待される有効性を満たしていますか？ 必要に応じて，AHU，水システム，圧縮空気／ガス，汚水／廃棄物の処理などの専用ユーティリティを用意していますか？ ユーティリティの逆流が交叉汚染のリスクの原因になる可能性はありますか？	
IV-30	Where starting and primary packaging materials, intermediate or bulk products are exposed to the environment, interior surfaces should be smooth, free from cracks and open joints, and should not shed particulate matter and should permit easy and effective cleaning and, if necessary, disinfection.	Do you design the premises to be ease of cleaning or decontamination e.g. to minimize collection points for powder that may be difficult to clean?	Part I - 3.9
	出発原料および一次包装材料，中間製品またはバルク製品が環境に暴露される場合は，建物内部の表面は，平滑でひび割れおよび開放接合部がなく，微粒子物質を脱落させないものであるとともに，容易かつ効果的な清掃および（必要な場合）消毒が行えるものであること	施設は，清掃または汚染除去を容易にするように設計していますか？ 例えば洗浄が難しい粉末が集まる場所などは？	
IV-31	Premises should preferably be laid out in such a way as to allow the production to take place in areas connected in a logical order corresponding to the sequence of the operations and to the requisite cleanliness levels.	Do you design wash rooms adequately to ensure they are not a risk of cross-contamination or recontamination?	Part I - 3.7
	作業の流れおよび必要な清浄度レベルに応じた論理的な順序で連結した区域において製造が行われるよう，建物を設計すること	洗浄室は交叉汚染や再汚染の危険性がないように適切に設計されていますか？	
IV-32	Production areas should be effectively ventilated, with air control facilities appropriate both to the products handled, to the operations undertaken within them and to the external environment.	Do you design the zoning and associated AHU to ensure pressure cascades and air flows to avoid cross contamination appropriately? Do you design air flows to take account of occurrences such as operation of local extract, vacuum transfer systems and doors opening?	Part I - 3.12
	製造区域は，取り扱う製品，そこで行われる作業および外部環境のいずれに対しても適切な空調設備を使用して，効果的に換気すること	区分け（ゾーニング），それに関連するAHUは，圧力勾配／カスケードおよびエアフローを確実にし，適切に交叉汚染を防止するよう設計されていますか？ 空気の流れは，局所的な抜け，真空搬送システム，ドアの開閉などが起きることを考慮して設計していますか？	
IV-33	In cases where dust is generated, specific provisions should be taken to avoid cross-contamination and facilitate cleaning.	Do you have appropriate local extraction of containment to control the spread of dust/vapors at source?	Part I - 3.12, 3.14
	じん埃が発生する場合は，交叉汚染を回避して清掃を行いやすくする特別な予防措置を講じること	じん埃／蒸気の発生源を管理するための適切な局所排出または封じ込めがありますか？	

チェック NO	PIC/S Requirement／PIC/Sの要求項目	Questions／監査時の質問例	PIC/S GMP Guide NO.
IV-34	The outcome of the Quality Risk Management process should be the basis for determining the extent of technical and organizational measures required to control risks for cross-contamination.	In the case AHU recirculation is used, do you have adequate controls for the filtration system to ensure that airborne contamination is removed? Is reliance on filtration in the AHU system appropriate for the hazard presented?	Part Ⅰ- 3.12, 5.21
	品質リスク管理プロセスの結果は，交叉汚染のリスクを管理するために必要な技術的および組織的手順の範囲を決定するための基礎となるべきである	AHUの再循環が行われている場合，フィルターシステムが空気中の汚染物質を確実に除去するのに適切な管理装置を備えていますか？ AHUシステムにおけるろ過の信頼性は，存在するハザードに適切ですか？	
IV-35	Lighting, temperature, humidity and ventilation should be appropriate and such that they do not adversely affect, directly or indirectly, either the medicinal products during their manufacture and storage, or the accurate functioning of equipment.	If the site operates a low power mode or switch off AHU out of hours could you assess, justify and demonstrate effectiveness (depending on the extent of the hazard) in controlling cross-contamination? • Has consideration been given to the impact during power down and power up or power failure? • Could there be any unintended consequences deviation (e.g. loss of containment or pressure reversal)? • Has the company documented an assessment for the time needed to return to a clean status once power is switched back on after power off / reduced power?	Part Ⅰ- 3.3, 3.12
	照明，温度，湿度および換気が適切でありそれらが製造および保管中の医薬品または装置の正確な作動に直接的または間接的に悪影響を及ぼさないこと	サイトが低消費電力モードで動作しているか，AHUを就業時間以外はオフにしている場合は，（ハザードの大きさによるが）交叉汚染管理の有効性が評価され，正当化されていますか？ 停電または電源事故の際の影響を考慮していますか？ 逸脱・意図しない結果（封じ込めや圧力の逆転など）がありますか？ 電圧低下・電源が切れた後に電源回復した際，クリーンな状態に戻るのに必要な時間の評価が文書化されていますか？	
IV-36	Layout and design must aim to minimize the risk of errors and permit effective cleaning and maintenance in order to avoid cross-contamination, build-up of dust or dirt and, in general, any adverse effect on the quality of products.	Do you have appropriate mechanisms to detect failure of control mechanisms, particularly where higher hazard products are manufactured (e.g. AHU failure)?	Part Ⅰ-3 principle
	配置および設計は，過誤のリスクを最小にすることを目途とするとともに，交叉汚染，じん埃または汚れの蓄積および製品品質への悪影響を回避するために，有効な洗浄および保守管理を可能とするものでなければならない	特にハザードの高い医薬品が製造される場合，管理機能の異常（AHUの故障など）を検知する適切なメカニズムを備えていますか？	

2 Premises, Equipment

チェック NO	PIC/S Requirement／PIC/Sの要求項目	Questions／監査時の質問例	PIC/S GMP Guide NO.
IV-37	Premises should be designed and equipped so as to afford maximum protection against the entry of insects or other animals.	Do you have appropriate design measures, in terms of equipment, for prevention of cross-contamination and are they consistent with the output of the QRM study? Does the qualification of the equipment support the cross-contamination control strategy and design philosophy?	Part I - 3.34, 1.6, Annex 15-3
	昆虫または他の動物の侵入を防ぐように建物を設計し，装備すること	交叉汚染の防止のために，機器の面で適切な設計措置を講じていますか？QRM試験の結果と一致していますか？装置の適格性は，交叉汚染制御戦略と設計思想をサポートしていますか？	
IV-38	Appropriate use of air-locks and pressure cascade to confine potential airborne contaminant within a specified area.	Where open processing is used (for dispensing, sampling), do you have appropriate controls and rationale?	Part I - 3.34, 5.20, 5.21
	特定区域内で潜在的な浮遊汚染物質を封じ込めるエアロックと圧力勾配の適切な使用	開放条件で作業が行われる場所・区域について，管理とその管理根拠は適切ですか？	
IV-39	Manufacturing equipment should be designed so that it can be easily and thoroughly cleaned.	Do you design the equipment to facilitate ease of cleaning and confirmation of cleanliness (e.g. visual inspection, swabbing)? Where cleanliness cannot be confirmed then, do you consider to use of dedicated equipment or parts?	Part I - 3.36, 5.21
	製造設備は，容易にかつ完全に清掃できるよう設計すること	洗浄と洗浄後の確認（例：目視検査，拭き取り）が容易になるように機器・装置が設計されていますか？清潔さが確認できない・困難な場所には，専用の機器や治具の使用が検討されていますか？	
IV-40	Washing and cleaning equipment should be chosen and used in order not to be a source of contamination.	If Clean In Place (CIP) or Clean out of Place (COP) systems (e.g. skids for vessel cleaning, or washing machines for parts) are utilized, do you design appropriately? Do you investigate that the systems are not to represent a potential for cross-contamination themselves?	Part I - 3.1, 3.37, Annex 15-3
	洗浄および清掃設備は，汚染源とならないよう選定し，使用すること	クリーンインプレース（CIP）システムまたはクリーンアウトオブプレース（COP）システム（例えば，容器・反応槽の洗浄のための滑材または部品のための洗濯機）が利用される場合，それらは適切に設計されていますか？システムが潜在的な交叉汚染源にならないことが確認されていますか？	
IV-41	All types of document should be defined and adhered to. The requirements apply equally to all forms of document media types.	Do you adequately identify difficulty to clean parts of equipment and is this supported by appropriate justification? Do you have a clear procedure to define how this should be conducted?	Part I - 3.37, 3.38, 4.1
	すべての種類の文書を規定し，遵守すること。要求事項は，すべての形態の文書の媒体形式に同様に適用する	機器の洗浄が困難な箇所を適切に識別しており，これは適切に正当化されていますか？これをどのように実施すべきかを定義する明確な手順はありますか？	

チェック NO	PIC/S Requirement／PIC/Sの要求項目	Questions／監査時の質問例	PIC/S GMP Guide NO.
IV-42	The outcome of the Quality Risk Management process should be the basis for determining the extent of technical and organizational measures required to control risks for cross-contamination.	Do you consider maintenance, In Process Control (IPC) and sampling (including equipment, personnel protective equipment/clothing, tools and change parts) as part of contamination control? Where appropriate, do you follow to control measures?	Part Ⅰ - 5.21
	品質リスク管理プロセスの結果は，交叉汚染のリスクを管理するために必要な技術的および組織的手順の範囲を決定するための基礎となるべきである	メンテナンス，工程内管理（IPC）およびサンプリング（機器，保護具／衣類，工具および交換部品を含む）は汚染管理の一部とみなされていますか？ 必要に応じて，管理手順が実施されていますか？	

3 General Organisational Controls / 一般組織管理

組織としての決め事

サンプリングや原料の取扱いなど，組織として適切な運用方法を規定し，それが遵守されているかを確認することとなる。リスクに応じた対応が求められるが，手順や記録があっても守られていなければ意味がない。

チェック NO	PIC/S Requirement／PIC/Sの要求項目	Questions／監査時の質問例	PIC/S GMP Guide NO.
IV-43	There should be periodic management review, with the involvement of senior management, of the operation of the Pharmaceutical Quality System to identify opportunities for continual improvement of products, processes and the system itself.	Where relevant, do you focus appropriate organizational controls to address risks identified in the risk assessment? Do you periodically review and/or up date your risk assessment?	Part I - 1.6, 5.19
	製品，工程およびシステム自体の継続的な改善の機会を特定するため，上級経営陣の関与の下，医薬品質システムの運用についての定期的マネジメントレビューがなされること	リスクアセスメントで特定されたリスクに対処するために，組織化された管理を実施していますか？ 定期的にリスクアセスメントの見直し，更新を行っていますか？	
IV-44	In cases where dust is generated (e.g. during sampling, weighing, mixing and processing operations, packaging of dry products), specific provisions should be taken to avoid cross-contamination and facilitate cleaning.	Do you preclean and/or protect contaminated equipment adequately before being moved to a general clean area?	Part I - 3.8, 3.14
	じん埃が発生する場合（例えば，サンプリング，秤量，混合および加工の作業中，乾いた状態の製品の包装時）は，交叉汚染を回避して清掃を行いやすくする特別な予防措置を講じること	一般的な洗浄区域に移動する前に，汚染された機器を適切に事前清掃および／または保護していますか？	
IV-45	The adequacy of the working and in-process storage space should permit the orderly and logical positioning of equipment and materials so as to minimize the risk of confusion between different medicinal products or their components, to avoid cross-contamination and to minimize the risk of omission or wrong application of any of the manufacturing or control steps.	Do you identify mobile or fixed equipment/accessories and ensure equipment status and secure to prevent mix up? Do you document the process adequately?	Part I - 3.8
	異なる医薬品またはその構成物の混同を最小化し，交叉汚染を回避，製造もしくは管理ステップの実施漏れ，または誤った適用のリスクを最小限にするよう，適切な作業スペースおよび工程内保管スペースに装置および物品を整然と配置すること	移動可能な機器または据え付け機器／付属品は識別されており，機器のステータスが明確にされ，混同防止が確実にされていますか？ プロセスは適切に文書化されていますか？	

チェック NO	PIC/S Requirement／PIC/Sの要求項目	Questions／監査時の質問例	PIC/S GMP Guide NO.
IV-46	Labels applied to containers, equipment or premises should be clear, unambiguous and in the company's agreed format. It is often helpful in addition to the wording on the labels to use colors to indicate status.	Do you clearly identify and/or label dedicated equipment/parts and control appropriately?	Part I - 5.13
	容器，装置または建物に適用する表示は，明瞭かつ明解であり，合意した書式であること。当該表示上の文言に加えて，状態を色分けして示すことは，多くの場合有用	専用の機器／部品には，適切な識別・ラベルと適切な管理がされていますか？	
IV-47	Testing methods should be validated. A laboratory that is using a testing method and which did not perform the original validation, should verify the appropriateness of the testing method.	Is your sampling program suitable to detect spread of contamination from a controlled area to verify that containment measures are effective?	Part I - 6.15
	試験方法をバリデートすること。元のバリデーションを実施していない試験方法を用いる試験室は，当該試験方法の適切性を検証すること	サンプリングプログラムは，封じ込め措置が有効であることを確認するために管理区域からの汚染の広がりを検出するのに適していますか？	
IV-48	Specific measures for waste handling, contaminated rinsing water and soiled gowning.	Do you have the control and monitoring measurement /procedures of effluent/waste streams adequate to control the risk of cross-contamination or recontamination from the waste stream, based on the level of hazard?	Part I - 1.12, 1.13, 5.21
	廃棄物処理，汚染されたすすぎ水および汚れた保護具のための特定の措置	ハザードのレベルに基づく，廃棄物の流れからの交叉汚染または再汚染のリスクを管理するのに適切な排水／廃棄物の流れ管理とモニタリング手順がありますか？	
IV-49	Where starting and primary packaging materials, intermediate or bulk products are exposed to the environment, interior surfaces should be smooth, free from cracks and open joints, and should not shed particulate matter and should permit easy and effective cleaning and, if necessary, disinfection.	In the case any time product or starting materials are exposed to the environment, do you control adequate to prevent cross-contamination?	Part I - 3.9, 5.20, 5.21
	出発原料および一次包装材料，中間製品またはバルク製品が環境中に暴露される場合は，建物内部の表面は，平滑でひび割れおよび開放接合部がなく，微粒子物質を脱落させないものであるとともに，容易かつ効果的な清掃および消毒が行えるものであること	製品または出発材料が環境中に暴露されるとき，交叉汚染を防止するのに十分な管理が行われていますか？	

チェック NO	PIC/S Requirement／PIC/Sの要求項目	Questions／監査時の質問例	PIC/S GMP Guide NO.
IV-50	Weighing of starting materials usually should be carried out in a separate weighing room designed for such use. Operations on different products should not be carried out simultaneously or consecutively in the same room unless there is no risk of mix-up or cross-contamination.	Do you adequately store and handle material to prevent cross-contamination and reflective of the material hazards? Are materials kept adequately sealed until point of use? Are sampling tools adequately cleaned, dedicated or disposable? Is the area where materials are sampled or dispensed adequately cleaned between different products?	Part Ⅰ - 3.1, 3.13, 3.18, 3.22, 3.24, 5.9, 5.11
	出発原料の秤量は通常，その用途のために設計され，区分された秤量室で行うこと。 異なる製品についての作業は，混同または交叉汚染のリスクが皆無である場合を除き，同じ作業室で同時に，または連続して行ってはならない	交叉汚染を防止し，原材料のハザードを反映させるために，原材料の保管と取り扱いは適切ですか？ 材料は使用時まで適切に封印されていますか？ サンプリングツールは適切に洗浄，専用化または使い捨てを採用できますか？ 異なる製品間で材料をサンプリング，または秤量・小分けする区域は適切に洗浄されていますか？	
IV-51	Storage areas should be of sufficient capacity to allow orderly storage of the various categories of materials and products: starting and packaging materials, intermediate, bulk and finished products, products in quarantine, released, rejected, returned or recalled.	Do you adequately store and handle material to prevent cross-contamination and reflective of the material hazards? Are arrangements for storage appropriate for the hazard? Is labelling adequately controlled to prevent mix up of materials?	Part Ⅰ - 3.18
	保管区域は，以下のようなさまざまなカテゴリーの原材料および製品を整然と保管できる十分な広さであること；出発物質および包装材料，中間品，バルク製品および最終製品，区分保管中の製品，合格判定された製品，不合格判定された製品，返品または回収された製品	交叉汚染や重大な危険を防ぐために，適切に保管して取り扱っていますか？ 災害に適した保管の手配はありますか？ 材料の混同を防ぐため，表示は適切に管理されていますか？	
IV-52	A state of control is established and maintained by developing and using effective monitoring and control systems for process performance and product quality. The results of product and processes monitoring are taken into account in batch release, in the investigation of deviations, and, with a view to taking preventive action to avoid potential deviations occurring in the future. Recording of spills, accidental events or deviations from procedures.	Do you have adequate systems to detect, record and assess impact of situations such as spillages or other unusual events that could lead to cross-contamination?	Part Ⅰ - 1.4, 5.21
	工程の能力および製品品質の効果的なモニタリングおよび管理のシステムを開発し，それを用いることによって，管理された状態を確立し，維持する。 バッチの出荷可否判定，逸脱の原因究明において，製品および工程のモニタリングの結果を考慮するとともに，将来発生する可能性がある逸脱を避ける予防措置の観点からも考慮する。 漏れ，偶発事象または手順からの逸脱を記録する	交叉汚染を引き起こす可能性のある漏出やその他の異常事態の影響を検出，記録，評価する適切なシステムを持っていますか？	

チェック NO	PIC/S Requirement／PIC/Sの要求項目	Questions／監査時の質問例	PIC/S GMP Guide NO.
IV-53	Premises should be situated in an environment which, when considered together with measures to protect the manufacture, presents minimal risk of causing contamination of materials or products. Premises should be carefully maintained, ensuring that repair and maintenance operations do not present any hazard to the quality of products Use of "closed systems" for processing and material/product transfer between equipment.	Do you have the equipment/facility subject to adequate preventative maintenance to prevent potential cross-contamination? For example, are there any issues with duct work or transfer line leaks that may contaminate other areas?	Part Ⅰ- 3.1, 3.2, 3.8, 3.10, 5.21
	製造を保護する手段と併せて考慮すると，原材料および製品の汚染を引き起こすリスクが最小限である環境に，建物があるべき。補修および保守管理の作業が製品の品質に危害をもたらさないことを保証するよう，建物を注意深く維持管理すること。製造と機器の間での材料／製品移送に「閉鎖系システム」を使用する	潜在的な交叉汚染を防止するために，装置／設備は適切な予防保守が施されていますか？たとえば，ダクトや他の区域を汚染する可能性のある移送ラインの漏れが起こる可能性はありますか？	
IV-54	Any activity covered by the GMP Guide that is outsourced should be appropriately defined, agreed and controlled in order to avoid misunderstandings which could result in a product or operation of unsatisfactory quality.	Do you assign any contract services providers (e.g. contract testing, contracted cleaning services, contract manufacture for other markets) that may introduce hazardous substances? If so, are they appropriately identified, assessed and controlled? Are contract service providers appropriately trained regarding control measures employed by the manufacturer? Are contract service providers appropriately qualified and certified after training?	Part Ⅰ-7 principle, 1.18
	GMPガイドラインがカバーする業務について外部委託する場合は，不適切な品質の製品または作業につながり得る誤解を回避するため，適正に定義し，関係者が同意し，管理すること	有害物質が混入する可能性のある外部契約業務サービス（委託試験，洗浄，CMOなど）は利用していますか？もしそうなら，（有害物質が混入する可能性を）適切に特定し，評価し，管理していますか？受託業者は，委託者が採用した管理手順・基準に関して適切な教育・訓練を受けていますか？教育・訓練後，認定されていますか？	

3 General Organisational Controls

チェックNO	PIC/S Requirement／PIC/Sの要求項目	Questions／監査時の質問例	PIC/S GMP Guide NO.
IV-55	Every person entering the manufacturing areas should wear protective garments appropriate to the operations to be carried out. The Pharmaceutical Quality System of the Contract Giver should include the control and review of any outsourced activities.	In the case in-house laundry practices, do you control internal laundry procedure and facilities to prevent-cross-contamination between different products? In the case external laundry contractors, do you ensure their appropriate controls to prevent cross-contamination with other manufacturer's products? Where appropriate, do you have any evidence and/or decontamination that processes applied would be effective?	Part I - 2.18, 7 principle, 7.3, 7.4, 7.6, 7.9
	製造区域に立ち入るすべての者は，実施する作業に応じた適切な保護衣を着用すること。 委託者の医薬品品質システムは，外部委託作業の管理および照査を含むこと	自社で作業着等を洗濯する場合，作業着等の洗濯とその施設を，異なる製品間の交叉汚染を防ぐために管理していますか？ 外部の洗濯業者の起用は，他の製造業者の製品との交叉汚染を防ぐために適切に管理を行っていますか？ 必要であるならば，除染プロセスが適用されており，効果的である証拠を有していますか？	

4 Campaign Manufacture Organisation/キャンペーン製造

リスクを最小化

製造区域における交叉汚染リスクを最小限度に抑えることが要件となる。共用施設を用いることなどもあると想定されるため，製造所において具体的にどのような対策が立てられているか，その対策が真に有効なものであるかをチェックする。

チェックNO	PIC/S Requirement／PIC/Sの要求項目	Questions／監査時の質問例	PIC/S GMP Guide NO.
IV-56	Dedicating the whole manufacturing facility or a self-contained production area on a campaign basis (dedicated by separation in time) followed by a cleaning process of validated effectiveness.	Do you have concreted overall strategy for campaign manufacture in shared facilities adequate to prevent cross contamination?	Part I - 5.20, 5.21
	全製造施設の専用化，またはキャンペーンベースで自己完結型の生産エリア（時間を隔てることによって専用化）はバリデートされた手法で洗浄する	共用施設を用いてのキャンペーン製造をする際，交叉汚染を防止する具体的かつ全体的な戦略を持っていますか？	
IV-57	The influence of the time between manufacture and cleaning and the time between cleaning and use should be taken into account to define dirty and clean hold times for the cleaning process. Where campaign manufacture is carried out, the impact on the ease of cleaning at the end of the campaign should be considered and the maximum length of a campaign should be the basis for cleaning validation exercises.	Do you adequately define dirty holding period with scientific sounds?	Annex 15-10.8, 10.9
	製造終了と洗浄開始までの時間，洗浄終了と再度使用開始までの時間の影響を考慮して，ダーティー／クリーン保持時間を定義する必要がある。キャンペーン製造が行われる場合，キャンペーン製造終了時の洗浄の容易・困難さを考慮し，キャンペーンの最大値を洗浄の実証の基礎とすべき	製造から洗浄開始までの時間を科学的根拠に基づいて定めていますか？	

4 Campaign Manufacture Organisation

チェックNO	PIC/S Requirement／PIC/Sの要求項目	Questions／監査時の質問例	PIC/S GMP Guide NO.
IV-58	Manufacturing equipment should be designed, located and maintained to suit its intended purpose. Repair and maintenance operations should not present any hazard to the quality of the products. Depending on the contamination risk, verification of cleaning of non-product contact surfaces and monitoring of air within the manufacturing area and/or adjoining areas in order to demonstrate effectiveness of control measures against airborne contamination or contamination by mechanical transfer.	Do you adequately minimize and/or reduce less than acceptable criteria the opportunities for cross-contamination of equipment in the processing area? Is equipment, that is not required for manufacture removed from the area? If movement of equipment is necessary is it confirmed clean and is the previous use of the equipment compatible with the location it will be moved to? Do you adequately protect, or re-clean afterwards, equipment that is not required for production but cannot be removed from the area? Is this appropriate for the nature of the product hazard? Is movement of ancillary equipment (e.g. IPC test equipment) and materials between campaigns (of different products) and areas adequately controlled?	Part Ⅰ-1.13, 3.34, 3.35, 5.21
	製造設備は，その目的に適するよう設計し，配置し，保守管理すること。 補修および保守管理の作業は，製品品質に危害をもたらしてはならない。 汚染の危険性に応じて，機械的な移送による汚染移動による空気汚染に対する管理措置の有効性を実証するために，非製品接触面の洗浄と製造エリアおよび／または隣接する区域内の空気のモニタリングを検証すること	製造区域内の機器の交叉汚染の可能性を適切に最小化もしくは基準以下にしていますか？ 製造に必要ではない機器が，その区域から取り除かれていますか？ 機器の移動が必要な場合は，それが清浄であることが確認され，移動先で元の仕様の互換性がありますか？ 製造業者は，生産のために必要ではないが，その区域から移動できない設備を適切に保全しているか，または後で再洗浄していますか？ これらの移動は製品ハザードの性質に適していますか？ 補助機器（IPC試験機器など）とキャンペーン（異なる製品の）と区域間の原材料の移動が適切に管理されていますか？	
IV-59	Premises should preferably be laid out in such a way as to allow the production to take place in areas connected in a logical order corresponding to the sequence of the operations and to the requisite cleanliness levels.	Do you have any adequate procedure to describe cleaning of non-product contact equipment such as phones, chairs, fire extinguishers, computer keyboards etc.?	Part Ⅰ-3.1, 3.2, 3.7, 3.9, 4.1
	作業の流れおよび必要な清浄度レベルに応じた論理的な順序で連結した区域において製造が行われるよう，建物を設計すること	製造・製品には直接関係しない機器（電話，椅子，消火器，コンピュータキーボードなど）の洗浄・清掃について記載した適切な手順はありますか？	

5 Equipment Cleaning／機器の洗浄

汚染源となり得るものを特定

製造に用いる機器が汚染源となることもある。そのため適切に清掃されているか，また清浄レベルを目視で確認する場合には適切に確認作業が行われているかがカギになる。

チェックNO	PIC/S Requirement／PIC/Sの要求項目	Questions／監査時の質問例	PIC/S GMP Guide NO.
IV-60	For all cleaning processes an assessment should be performed to determine the variable factors which influence cleaning effectiveness and performance. If variable factors have been identified, the worst-case situations should be used as the basis for cleaning validation studies.	Do you have any procedures for developing the cleaning methods of equipment that requires adequate assessment, detail and evidence (i.e. are use of equipment drawings, equipment manufacturers manual and physical examination of equipment specified)? Do you have cleaning instructions with the level of detail in reflect the hazard level and reflect the complexity of equipment? for example: ・Are all variables specified in adequate detail? ・Has an appropriate cleaning agent been selected? ・Is the concentration and other relevant parameters such as contact time of the cleaning agent specified? ・Are areas hard to clean clearly specified? ・Is control of cleaning equipment and re-use of cleaning equipment (e.g. mop handles) specified? Are records of cleaning adequate to reflect the level of control required?	Annex 15-10, Part Ⅰ-4.1, 4.3, 4.4
	すべての洗浄プロセスについて，洗浄の有効性および性能に影響を与える変動因子を決定するための評価が行われなければならない。変動要因が特定されている場合は，洗浄バリデーションの根拠としてワーストケースで行うべき	洗浄効果の適切な評価，詳細および証拠が求められる機器の洗浄方法を開発する手順がありますか（すなわち，機器図面，機器メーカーのマニュアルおよび特定の機器の物理的検査の使用に関するもの）？ 洗浄指示書は，ハザードレベル，機器の複雑さを反映して，それ相応の詳細さで準備されていますか？たとえば； ・すべての変数が適切に規格化されていますか？ ・適切な洗浄剤が選択されていますか？ ・洗浄剤の接触時間，濃度およびその他の関連パラメータが規格化されていますか？ ・清浄が難しい区域は，明確に特定されていますか？ ・洗浄器具の管理と洗浄器具（モップハンドルなど）の再使用は標準化されていますか？ 必要な管理レベルを十分反映した掃除記録がありますか？	
IV-61	Premises should be carefully maintained, ensuring that repair and maintenance operations do not present any hazard to the quality of products.	Do you define that the equipment cleaning coordinate with area cleaning to prevent re-contamination?	Part Ⅰ-3.1, 3.2

5 Equipment Cleaning

チェック NO	PIC/S Requirement／PIC/Sの要求項目	Questions／監査時の質問例	PIC/S GMP Guide NO.
IV-61	補修および保守管理の作業が製品の品質に危害をもたらさないことを保証するよう，建物を注意深く維持管理すること	再汚染を防ぐために，機器のクリーニングとエリアクリーニングを同等とすることを定義していますか？	
IV-62	Validation should consider the level of automation in the cleaning process. Where an automatic process is used, the specified normal operating range of the utilities and equipment should be validated.	Do you adequately define the level of preparation/dismantling of equipment required with manual cleaning, COP and CIP processes for consistent application?	Annex 15-10.4, Part I - 1.12, 1.13, 4.3, 4.4,
	バリデーションでは，洗浄プロセスにおける自動化のレベルを考慮する必要がある。自動洗浄プロセスが使用される場合，ユーティリティおよび装置の特定の正常な動作範囲がバリデートされるべき	一貫した適用のために手動洗浄，COPおよびCIPプロセスに必要な設備の準備／解体のレベルを適切に定義していますか？	
IV-63	Documents containing instructions should be laid out in an orderly fashion and be easy to check.	Do you have any figures, diagrams or photographs depicting dismantled equipment used to support consistency and error proofing of cleaning?	Part I - 4.4
	指図書を含む文書は，整頓して配置し，チェックしやすくすること	洗浄の不備の検証や一致に役立つ，分解した機器の図面や写真はありますか？	
IV-64	Specific measures for waste handling, contaminated rinsing water and soiled gowning; Drains should be of adequate size and have trapped gullies. Open channels should be avoided where possible, but if necessary, they should be shallow to facilitate cleaning and disinfection.	Do you control effluent and waste from the cleaning process in a manner that does not allow cross-contamination or re-contamination?	Part I - 3.11, 5.21
	排水溝は，適切なサイズで，トラップ付きの落とし込みを有すること。開放溝は可能な限り避けるが，必要であれば，清掃および消毒を実施しやすいよう浅くしておくこと	洗浄プロセスからの排水と廃棄物を，交叉汚染や再汚染をしないように管理していますか？	
IV-65	A visual check for cleanliness is an important part of the acceptance criteria for cleaning validation. It is not generally acceptable for this criterion alone to be used.	Do you have the specification and/or procedure of visual inspection for cleanliness of equipment to control and verify? Where visual inspection of closed process equipment is not possible at each turnaround, has the cleanliness of the equipment and transfer lines been adequately proven during validation? Do you have the visual inspection process, where applicable, to describe and conduct in a manner to ensure that potential contaminants will be seen? Do you have adequate justification where visual inspection cannot be conducted?	Annex 15-10.2
	清浄度の目視検査は，洗浄のバリデーションの合格基準の重要な部分である。一般的には，この基準のみを使用することは認められない	機器の清浄の検証・管理のための目視検査の規格・プロセスは準備されていますか？ 定期検査で閉鎖型製造装置の目視検査が不可能な場合，バリデーション中に装置および移送ラインの清浄性が十分に証明されていますか？ 目視検査プロセスは，潜在的な汚染物質が確実に検出できるように明確に文書化され，実施されていますか？ 目視検査が行えない場合，適切な検証を行っていますか？	

チェックNO	PIC/S Requirement／PIC/Sの要求項目	Questions／監査時の質問例	PIC/S GMP Guide NO.
IV-66	For all cleaning processes an assessment should be performed to determine the variable factors which influence cleaning effectiveness and performance. All necessary facilities for GMP are provided including; • Appropriately qualified and trained personnel.	Do you qualify visual inspectors with proper criteria to find meaningful amount of residual under condition defined procedure? Do you have appropriate methods and tools to help detect residues by visual inspection (e.g. use of a good light or mirror) adequately defined by procedure?	Part I - 1.8, 2.10, 2.11, Annex 15-10.2, 10.5
	すべての洗浄プロセスについて，洗浄の有効性および性能に影響を与える変動因子を決定するための評価が行われなければならない。 以下を含む，GMPに必要なすべての施設を備えていること ・適切に適格性が確認され，教育訓練された人員	目視検査実施者は，手順書に記載された残留限界を検出できることを認定されていますか？ 適切に定義された目視検査（例えば，良好な光源または鏡の使用）によって残留物を検出するのに役立つ方法およびツールが使用されていますか？	
IV-67	Production and control operations are clearly specified and Good Manufacturing Practice adopted.	Is the person conducting the final visual inspection adequately independent of the cleaning operation?	Part I - 1.4
	製造および管理の作業を明確に規定し，GMPを適用する	最終目視検査を実施する者は，洗浄作業者とは適切に独立していますか？	
IV-68	Checks that the equipment and work station are clear of previous products, documents or materials not required for the planned process, and that equipment is clean and suitable for use.	Do you verify line clearance to ensure that any potential cross-contamination sources have been removed?	Part I - 4.18
	装置および作業台に以前の製品，行おうとする工程に不要な文書または原材料がないこと，ならびに装置が清掃され使用に適していることのチェック	潜在的な交叉汚染源の除去を確実にするために，ラインクリアランスが効果的に確認されていますか？	
IV-69	The results of product and processes monitoring are taken into account in batch release, in the investigation of deviations, and, with a view to taking preventive action to avoid potential deviations occurring in the future.	Do you have a system (e.g. deviation system) to record failures in cleaning such as: - Where execution of the prescribed cleaning instructions has failed to render the equipment clean - Where, upon, visual inspection by the independent person, the equipment is found to not be clean - When swab/rinse sample failures occur?	Part I - 1.4
	バッチの出荷可否判定，逸脱の原因究明において，製品および工程のモニタリングの結果を考慮するとともに，将来発生する可能性がある逸脱を避ける予防措置の観点からも考慮する	次のような洗浄の失敗を記録するシステム（例えば，逸脱システム）を有していますか？ ・規定の洗浄指示書を実施したが，装置の洗浄に失敗した場合 ・独立した担当者による目視検査の際に，装置が清潔でないことが判明した場合 ・スワブ／すすぎサンプルの失敗	

Cleaning Validation and Verification／洗浄バリデーション・ベリフィケーション

汚染防止の重点項目

製造設備の洗浄バリデーションは，交叉汚染防止対策の上で重点項目である。洗浄プロセスが，潜在するハザードに対して適切な方法であることが検証され，また洗浄頻度もリスクに応じて適切に定められている必要がある。また，昨今では毒性学的評価に基づく洗浄バリデーションの実施が求められている。より高いレベルでの運用が必要になってきている。

チェックNO	PIC/S Requirement／PIC/Sの要求項目	Questions／監査時の質問例	PIC/S GMP Guide NO.
IV-70	Cleaning validation should be performed in order to confirm the effectiveness of any cleaning procedure for all product contact equipment.	Do you validate the cleaning process and periodically verify the cleaning process in the appropriate manner and frequency required for the hazard presented?	Annex 15-10.1
	洗浄のバリデーションは，機器に接触するすべての製品の洗浄手順の有効性を確認するために行う必要がある	洗浄プロセスはバリデートされ，存在する危害に適切な方法と頻度で定期的に検証されていますか？	
IV-71	For all cleaning processes an assessment should be performed to determine the variable factors which influence cleaning effectiveness and performance.	Do you define the validation protocol in line an adequate structured approach to completing cleaning validation? In the case cleaning verification is used after each cleaning process, following or as part of the concurrent cleaning validation program, could you ensure that the equipment has been demonstrated to be clean prior to further use?	Part Ⅰ-1.4, Annex 15-10.5
	すべての洗浄プロセスについて，洗浄の有効性および性能に影響を与える変動因子を決定するための評価が行われなければならない	バリデーションプロトコールは，洗浄バリデーションを完了するための十分なアプローチを定義していますか？ 洗浄ベリフィケーションが各洗浄工程の後，または同時に行われる洗浄バリデーションプログラムの一環として，またはその一部として採用される場合，その後製造使用する前に清浄であることが十分に証明されていますか？	
IV-72	Where manual cleaning of equipment is performed, it is especially important that the effectiveness of the manual process should be confirmed at a justified frequency.	In the case manual cleaning is conducted, do you demonstrate the validation a that this manual method can be consistently applied by personnel? If the cleaning process is manual, do you verify/validate the reliability and effectiveness of the cleaning process confirmed through appropriate periodic verification?	Part Ⅰ-1.4, Annex 15-10.15
	機器の手動清掃を行う場合は，手作業の有効性を正当な頻度で確認すること	手作業による洗浄が行われている場合，この方法が担当者によって一貫して適用されることが適切に実証されていますか？ 洗浄プロセスが手動である場合，適切な定期的な検証を通じて洗浄プロセスの信頼性と有効性が確認されていますか？	

第IV章 Audit Checklist on Prevention for Cross Contamination／交叉汚染対策のためのチェックリスト

チェックNO	PIC/S Requirement／PIC/Sの要求項目	Questions／監査時の質問例	PIC/S GMP Guide NO.
IV-73	Limits for the carryover of product residues should be based on a toxicological evaluation.	Do you have the criteria for the carryover of product residues established based on toxicological evaluation and justified by risk assessment?	Part I - 1.4, Annex 15-10.6
	前製造からのキャリーオーバーの残留基準は，毒性学的評価に基づくものでなければならない	毒物学的評価に基づいて確立され，リスク評価によって正当化される製品残留物のキャリーオーバーの限度値は定められていますか？	
IV-74	Validation should consider the level of automation in the cleaning process. Where an automatic process is used, the specified normal operating range of the utilities and equipment should be validated.	Is the consistency and effectiveness of the automated cleaning process qualified and the methods validated? Have all variables and opportunities for malfunction (failure modes) of validated automated cleaning methods been identified, monitored and mitigated?	Part I - 1.4, Annex 15-10.4
	バリデーションでは，洗浄プロセスにおける自動化のレベルを考慮する必要がある。自動洗浄プロセスが使用される場合，ユーティリティおよび装置の特定の正常な動作範囲がバリデートされるべき	自動洗浄プロセスの一貫性と有効性が確認され，方法がバリデートされていますか？ バリデートされた自動洗浄方法の誤動作（故障モード）のためのすべての変数と条件が特定され，監視され，是正されていますか？	
IV-75	Recording of spills, accidental events or deviations from procedures.	Have all variables and opportunities for failure in manual cleaning and verification been identified, monitored and mitigated?	Part I - 5.21
	漏れ，偶発事象または手順からの逸脱を記録する	手作業での洗浄や調査の失敗のすべての変数と機会を特定，監視，是正していますか？	
IV-76	Written procedures should be in place to describe the actions to be taken if a planned change is proposed to a starting material, product component, process, equipment, premises, product range, method of production or testing, batch size, design space or any other change during the lifecycle that may affect product quality or reproducibility.	Are changes to any cleaning processes adequately assessed and recorded for impact on cleaning validation/verification?	Annex 15-11.2
	製品の品質や再現性に影響を与える可能性のあるライフサイクルでの変更（出発材料，製品構成物，プロセス，設備，施設，製品規格幅，製造方法または試験方法，バッチサイズ，設計スペースまたはその他）に関して，計画変更が提案された場合に実行される変更管理の手順書が準備されていること	洗浄プロセスの変更は洗浄のバリデーション／ベリフィケーションに与える影響について，適切に評価され記録されていますか？	
IV-77	Quality risk management is a systematic process for the assessment, control, communication and review of risks to the quality of the medicinal product. Processes and procedures should undergo periodic critical re-validation to ensure that they remain capable of achieving the intended results.	Is the type of revalidation or ongoing verification frequency appropriate and has a sound scientific rationale been applied? Are all deviations related to cleaning investigated and taken into consideration during the periodic review of cleaning validation/verification?	Part I - 1.12, 5.21, 5.26, Annex 15-11.7
	品質リスクマネジメントは，医薬品の品質へのリスク評価，管理，伝達および照査のための体系的なプロセスである。工程および手順が意図された結果を達成できることを保証するため，定期的にクリティカルな再バリデーションを行うこと	再バリデーションのタイプまたは継続中のベリフィケーションの頻度が適切であり，科学的根拠が適切に適用されていますか？ 洗浄のバリデーション／ベリフィケーションの定期的なレビュー中に，洗浄に関するすべての逸脱が調査され，考慮されていますか？	

チェックNO	PIC/S Requirement／PIC/Sの要求項目	Questions／監査時の質問例	PIC/S GMP Guide NO.
IV-78	If it is not feasible to test for specific product residues, other representative parameters may be selected. 特定の製品残留物を分析することができない場合は，他の代表的なパラメータを採用できる	In the case visual inspection of equipment, or parts of equipment (e.g. closed systems or pipework), is not possible at routine turnaround, could you have other methods of assuring cleanliness such as a validated rinse method? 機器や設備の部品（例えば，閉鎖システムや配管設備）の目視検査が日常的な処理では不可能な場合は，有効なすすぎ方法などの清浄性を保証する他の方法がありますか？	Annex 15-10.1, 10.2, 10.6
IV-79	A visual check for cleanliness is an important part of the acceptance criteria for cleaning validation. 清浄度の目視検査は，洗浄のバリデーションの合格基準の重要な部分である	Do you implement visual inspection in line with the complexity of the equipment and its potential to retain residue? 機器の複雑さと潜在的な残留物を考慮して目視検査を実施していますか？	Annex 15-10.1, 10.2.
IV-80	All necessary facilities for GMP are provided including: - Appropriately qualified and trained personnel; 以下を含む，GMPに必要なすべての施設を備えていること。 ・適切に適格性が確認され，教育訓練された人員	Do you qualify the personnel who perform swabbing as having the skills, knowledge and competency (recorded data and practical assessment) to ensure consistent application of the swabbing technique in accordance with the procedure? スワブを行う担当者は，スワブ手法をその手順に従って定量的に行うために，スキル，知識および能力（記録されたデータおよび実用的な評価）を有すると認定されていますか？	Part Ⅰ- 1.8, 2.10, 2.11
IV-81	Sampling should be carried out by swabbing and/or rinsing or by other means depending on the production equipment. The sampling materials and method should not influence the result. Recovery should be shown to be possible from all product contact materials sampled in the equipment with all the sampling methods used. サンプリングは，製造機器に応じて，スワブおよび／またはリンスまたは他の手段によって行うべきである。サンプリング材料および方法は，結果に影響を与えるべきではない。添加回収試験は，使用されるサンプリング方法で機器内すべての製品接触材料からサンプリング可能であることを示すこと	Do you appropriately validate analytical method for confirming that product residue has been removed in line with the acceptance criteria? Do you verify the recovery of swab and rinse samples? Are the values appropriate ones for the hazard? 合格基準に沿って製品残留物が除去されたことを確認するための，バリデートされた分析方法はありますか？ スワブおよびリンスサンプルの添加・回収率は適切に設定されていますか？ ハザードに対して，その値は適切ですか？	Annex 15-10.12

7 Personnel, Training／従業員・教育訓練

従業員教育の重要性

製造現場において，実際に作業を行う人員の教育は重要である。手順の不遵守などによって交叉汚染が起きてしまうことのないよう，従業員がGMPと品質リスクについての意識を持ちながら，製造業務にあたることが必須となる。

チェック NO	PIC/S Requirement／PIC/Sの要求項目	Questions／監査時の質問例	PIC/S GMP Guide NO.
IV-82	The manufacturer should provide training for all the personnel whose duties take them into production and storage areas or into control laboratories, and for other personnel whose activities could affect the quality of the product.	Do you adequately train personnel been trained and periodically assess them in processes to prevent cross-contamination and recontamination?	Part I - 2.10, 2.11
	製造業者は，職責により製造区域および保管区域または管理試験室に立ち入るすべての人員（技術，保守管理および清掃の人員を含む），およびその行動が製品品質に影響を及ぼす可能性のある他の人員に，教育訓練を実施すること	交叉汚染や再汚染防止のためのプロセスでは，人員を適切に訓練し，定期的に評価していますか？	
IV-83	Besides the basic training on the theory and practice of the Pharmaceutical Quality System and Good Manufacturing Practice, newly recruited personnel should receive training appropriate to the duties assigned to them.	Do you have any working requirement for personnel, to prevent opportunities for cross-contamination, defined in procedures and aligned to the hazard presented? Do you ensure that procedures/requirements are implemented and demonstrated to be effective?	Part I - 2.10, 2.11, 2.14, 4.1
	医薬品品質システムならびにGMPの理論および実践に関する基本的な教育訓練以外に，新規に採用された人員は，割り当てられた職責に応じた適切な教育訓練を受けること	存在する危害に合わせて定義された手順で，交叉汚染の機会を防止するための作業員の必要な行動要求はありますか？ 手順／要求項が実施され，有効であることが実証されていますか？	
IV-84	Supervision of working behavior to ensure training effectiveness and compliance with the relevant procedural controls.	Do you properly supervise or oversee processing areas to ensure that the personnel requirements are implemented to prevent opportunities for cross-contamination?	Part I - 2.10, 2.11, 2.14, 5.21
	トレーニングの有効性を確認し，関連する手順を遵守するための作業行動の監督	交叉汚染のきっかけを防ぐために必要な要員の要求項が確実に行われるように，適切な管理や監督が行われていますか？	
IV-85	Facilities for changing clothes and for washing and toilet purposes should be easily accessible and appropriate for the number of users.	Do you have properly change area and adequate clothing requirements (dress code) to prevent cross-contamination for all personnel that may enter and exit manufacturing areas?	Part I - 3.1, 3.31
	更衣設備ならびに手洗いおよびトイレ設備は，容易にアクセスでき，使用者数に対し適切な数があること	製造エリアに出入りする可能性のあるすべての人員の交叉汚染を防止するために，すべての更衣／服装要件は適切ですか？	

チェックNO	PIC/S Requirement／PIC/Sの要求項目	Questions／監査時の質問例	PIC/S GMP Guide NO.
IV-86	Washing and cleaning equipment should be chosen and used in order not to be a source of contamination. 洗浄および清掃機器は，汚染源とならないよう選定し，使用すること	Do you control the cleaning of protective clothing in a manner to prevent cross-contamination? 保護服の洗浄は交叉汚染を防止する方法で管理されていますか？	Part Ⅰ - 3.37, 5.21
IV-87	Keeping specific protective clothing inside areas where products with high risk of cross-contamination are processed. 交叉汚染のリスクが高い製品が製造される区域内では，特定の防護服を着用（保管）すること	Do you adequately control the re-use of Personal Protective Equipment (PPE) to protect it from recontamination and to prevent this being a source of cross-contamination? 個人用保護具（PPE）の再使用は再汚染から適切に保護し，交叉汚染の原因となるのを防ぐように管理されていますか？	Part Ⅰ - 5.21
IV-88	Steps should be taken in order to prevent the entry of unauthorized people. Production, storage and quality control areas should not be used as a right of way by personnel who do not work in them. 無許可の人の立入りを防止する方策が講じられていること。製造，保管および品質管理区域は，そこで作業しない人員が通路として使用してはならない	Do you control the movement of people, between production areas and/or between production and general area, to prevent cross-contamination in accordance with risk management principles? 生産区域間の人の移動は，リスク管理の原則に従って交叉汚染を防止するように管理されていますか？	Part Ⅰ - 1.12, 1.13, 3.5, 3.27, 5.21

日本語索引

アクション・アラート・レベル 58

アラームシステム 114, 120, 123, 135

逸脱 5, 14, 21, 26, 38, 71, 85, 113, 147, 160, 174

エンドトキシン 63, 65, 116

機器の洗浄 13, 126, 161, 170

機器の保守点検 13, 77

キャリーオーバー 29, 40, 174

休憩室 73, 77

教育訓練 6, 54, 72, 103, 132, 153, 155, 172, 175

供給業者 23, 89

局方 40, 130

空調システム 112

経営層 3, 5, 70, 72, 163

計量 26, 75, 85, 114

校正 13, 20, 79, 93, 114, 117, 120, 124, 135, 143

コロニー 143

コンサルタント 7

コンピュータ化システム 14

再サンプリング 131, 139

細胞バンク 58, 63

サンプリング 25, 27, 34, 57, 76, 81, 86, 89, 95, 130, 147, 163, 175

サンプリング室 76

サンプリング要員 132

残留基準 13, 40, 152, 174

時間制限 18, 27, 57

試験室管理記録 20

自己点検 4, 70, 103

試薬 20, 96, 129, 144

収率 19, 26

出荷判定 3, 19, 20, 32, 85, 90, 139

出発物質 2, 17, 75, 89, 108, 114, 131

照明 10, 160

生産部門 4, 21

セファロスポリン 9

洗浄記録 17

洗浄バリデーション 39, 151, 170, 173

チャレンジテスト（チャレンジ試験）
.... 9, 114, 117, 120

データの完全性 124

動線 8, 77, 118

トレーサビリティ 30, 33, 51, 59, 85, 129

バイオバーデン 63, 65, 120, 146

廃棄物 10, 108, 129, 159, 164, 171

排水 56, 75, 108, 115, 164, 171

バックアップ 15, 59, 120

バッチ製造記録 20

バッチ製造指示書 19

バリデーション基準 37

微生物学的 35, 97, 105, 123, 133

標準物質 125, 129

微粒子 114, 120, 143, 159, 162

品質照査 5, 39, 47, 71

品質部門 4, 18, 21, 28, 32, 34, 42,
                           72, 90, 96, 99, 137

品質リスクマネジメント 3, 71, 153, 174

封じ込め 9, 55, 107, 118, 155, 158, 161, 160

不純物プロファイル 29, 35, 38, 43

プロセスバリデーション 38

文書システム 16

閉鎖系システム 105, 166

ペニシリン 9, 75

ベントフィルター 60, 117

包装材料 17, 30, 34, 90, 159, 164

保管サンプル 36, 131, 135

マスター製造指示書 18

水処理システム 116

目視検査 171, 175

ユーザー要求仕様書 77

ラベル 11, 17, 26, 31, 34, 51, 76,
                           85, 87, 90, 96, 131, 164

リスクアセスメント 8, 13, 40, 157, 163

連続生産 13, 86

英語索引

Action and alert level 58

air conditional system 112

alarm system 58, 114, 117, 120, 135

back-up 15, 59, 120

batch production records 19, 85

bioburden 63, 65, 120, 146

calibration 13, 20, 93, 114, 117, 120, 124, 128, 142

carryover 29, 40, 152, 174

cell bank 58, 63

cephalosporin 9

cleaning validation 39, 62, 66, 151, 168, 170, 173

closed systems 105, 166, 175

computerized systems 14

consultants 7

containment 9, 55, 107, 118, 155, 158, 160, 164

continuous production 13, 86

deviation 5, 14, 21, 26, 38, 71, 84, 90, 113, 121, 147, 160, 165, 172, 174

endotoxin 63, 65, 116

equipment cleaning 17, 126, 130, 161, 170

equipment maintenance 13

HEPA filter 114, 142

high sensitive 9, 92

HVAC 55, 57, 107, 114

impurity profile 29, 35, 38, 43

internal audits 4, 70

LAF 57, 112

lighting 10, 160

OOS 5, 20, 34, 43, 71, 84, 90, 117, 138, 156

packaging materials 17, 30, 34, 41, 76, 81, 85, 90, 159, 164

particle 120, 143, 156

penicillin 9, 75	sampling room 76
Personnel for Sampling 132	self inspection 4, 70, 103
Pharmacopoeia 40, 133	starting materials 2, 75, 89, 108, 114
PQR 5, 47, 71, 102	supplier 22, 89, 95
process validation 38	
production activities 4, 10	time limits 27
	traceability 29, 33, 51, 59, 128
qualification 14, 38, 58, 113, 119, 125, 143, 158	training 6, 48, 54, 72, 103, 132, 153, 155, 166, 176
quality risk management 3, 71, 153, 162, 174	
quality unit 4, 18, 21, 28, 32, 34, 42, 90, 96, 99, 136	URS 77, 125
	validation policy 37
reagent 20, 96, 128	vent filters 60, 116
refreshment rooms 77	visual check 171, 175
responsibility of management 70	warter treatment 115
retention samples 36	weighing 26, 75, 163
risk assessment 8, 13, 38, 40, 63, 88, 90, 150, 157, 163, 175	yield 19, 26
sampling 27, 34, 57, 76, 81, 86, 89, 95, 130, 147, 163, 175	

著者略歴

古澤 久仁彦（ふるざわ くにひこ）

1978年住友化学工業に入社。農薬の創薬，安全性評価・開発登録等に従事。
2004年に三井農林に入社しAPIの製造部門にてFDA対応等を歴任。
2010年からテバ製薬の信頼性保証部門にてGMPコンプライアンス・グローバルGMP監査を担当。2014年退社。
その後フリーランスのGMPコンサルタントとして活動。

日英対訳 GMP監査チェックリスト
PIC/S GMPに基づく国内外製造所監査の勘所

定価　本体4,800円（税別）

2018年9月25日　　発　行
2021年4月30日　　第2刷発行

著　者　　古澤 久仁彦
発行人　　武田 正一郎
発行所　　株式会社 じほう
　　　　　101-8421　東京都千代田区神田猿楽町1-5-15（猿楽町SSビル）
　　　　　電話　編集 03-3233-6361　販売 03-3233-6333
　　　　　振替　00190-0-900481
　　　　　〈大阪支局〉
　　　　　541-0044　大阪市中央区伏見町2-1-1（三井住友銀行高麗橋ビル）
　　　　　電話　06-6231-7061

©2018　　　　　　　組版　(株)シンクス　　印刷　(株)日本制作センター
Printed in Japan

本書の複写にかかる複製，上映，譲渡，公衆送信（送信可能化を含む）の各権利は株式会社じほうが管理の委託を受けています。

JCOPY ＜出版者著作権管理機構 委託出版物＞
本書の無断複製は著作権法上での例外を除き禁じられています。
複製される場合は，そのつど事前に，出版者著作権管理機構（電話 03-5244-5088，FAX 03-5244-5089，e-mail：info@jcopy.or.jp）の許諾を得てください。

万一落丁，乱丁の場合は，お取替えいたします。
ISBN 978-4-8407-5120-9